Comments on **Alzheimer's and ot**
fingertips from readers and review

'For carers and families, this book provides a fount of knowledge and
experience that will be invaluable on the journey through dementia. Its
comprehensiveness and clarity ensure it is accessible and excellent value.'

NEIL HUNT,
mer's Society

'When I was mysel   his book
and realised that I w   lit   ank you.'

RACHEL CANNING,
Cornwall

'The advice to carers who ar   nt of deciding it is time to
think about a nursing home i   t on.'

FREDERIKA STRADLING,
whose mother has dementia, Wiltshire

'A very easy and informative r   lay person.'

MRS C S WATSON,
Hampshire

'The authors, all of whom have a thorough understanding of dementia,
have addressed almost every issue which could crop up in a day-to-day
caring situation and provided well-judged and practical answers.'

Living with Dementia

'. . . it's a veritable bible for sufferer and carer alike.'

RUSSELL GRANT
Daily Mail

Reviews of previous editions of **Alzheimer's and other Dementias:**
Answers at your fingertips

'. . . will certainly help anyone whose life has been touched by Alzheimer's. In
question-and-answer format, it covers every aspect of the disease's effects . . .'

BERNICE DAVIDSON,
Evening Standard

'. . . equally valuable reading for home carers and professionals. It is
written in simple language that is easily digested and understood.'

Alzheimer's News, New Zealand

'This book is for the superb loving carers of those suffering from Alzheimer's, and for anyone who wants to help them. Written in a question-and-answer format, it is the most practical guide you can imagine. It deals with every aspect of the condition, from its symptoms to its effects on daily life, ranging from legal and financial implications to coping with sexual needs to loneliness. It cannot be recommended too highly to those who need it – and to those who don't but could benefit from knowledge of the disease.'

CLAIRE RAYNER,
Mail on Sunday

Comments on previous editions of *Alzheimer's and other Dementias: Answers at your fingertips* from readers

'Absolutely invaluable – many thanks.'

MRS C NORTON
Devon

'It is a wonderful compendium of questions that are so often asked . . . I have read many books on Alzheimer's and I must say I believe this is the most practical one that I have seen.'

JEROME H. STONE, Founder and Honorary Vice President
of Alzheimer's Disease International, Founder of the Alzheimer's Association (USA)
and a former carer

'. . . a book which I am certain will become a bible for the ever-increasing number of people who have Alzheimer problems in the family.'

KATIE BOYLE

'. . . needed to be written, and could scarcely have been better done . . . nothing is too technical to have daunted the authors, all is simplified without distortion, and where there is uncertainty it is not hidden, but an honest judgement is offered.'

PROFESSOR TOM ARIE, CBE, MA, BM, FRCPsych, FFPHM, RASA,
Age Care

Alzheimer's and other Dementias

Answers at your fingertips

Harry Cayton OBE, BA, BPhil, DipAnth, FRSA, FFPH
Chief Executive, Council for Healthcare Regulatory Excellence
former Chief Executive, Alzheimer's Society UK

Dr Nori Graham BM BCh, FRCPsych, DUniv
Emeritus Consultant in Old Age Psychiatry,
Royal Free Hospital, London
former Chairman of Alzheimer's Disease International

Dr James Warner BSc, MB BS, MD,
MRCP(UK), MRCPsych, FHEA
Consultant in Older Adults Psychiatry, St Charles Hospital, London
Honorary Senior Lecturer in Old Age Psychiatry,
Imperial College London

CLASS PUBLISHING · LONDON

Printing history
First published 1997, reprinted 1998
Reprinted with revisions 1998
Second edition 2002, reprinted 2004
Third edition 2008, reprinted 2008, reprinted 2010

The authors and publisher welcome feedback from the users of this book. Please contact the publisher:

Class Publishing, Barb House, Barb Mews, London W6 7PA, UK
Telephone: 020 7371 2119
Fax: 020 7371 2878 [International +4420]
email: post@class.co.uk
Website: www.class.co.uk

A CIP catalogue for this book is available from the British Library.

ISBN 978 1 85959 148 2

10 9 8 7 6 5 4 3

Edited by Gillian Clarke
Cartoons by Linda Moore
Index by Vicki Robinson

Designed and typeset by Martin Bristow

Printed and bound in Gateshead by Athenaeum Press

Contents

Foreword

by **Tony Robinson**
actor, writer and tv presenter

This is a book for people with dementia, their families, carers and friends. We know that there are now 24 million people world-wide with Alzheimer's disease or one of the other dementias. Every one of them has a personal story to tell and faces similar difficulties and experiences. Each of them needs information and help throughout the course of the illness.

I've experienced dementia in my family and I know first-hand the benefit of sharing emotions and ideas with others and the value of straightforward information and advice.

That's where this book is so helpful. Based on real questions asked by people with dementia and their carers, it distils the wisdom and the experience of many people who have lived through the difficulties that dementia brings. It is packed with practical tips and honest, common-sense answers. The way the book is arranged means you can dip into it as and when you want and quickly find the answer to the problem you have at that time.

The authors of this book have many years of experience of looking after people with dementia and helping their families and carers. They understand the difficulties you may face and but also how you can find solutions to your problems. Since its first publication this book has become an essential guide for all those involved in caring for people with dementia and the people advising them. I recommend it heartily!

Acknowledgements

In preparing the third edition of this book we have drawn on our own experience and reading, and are grateful to all our colleagues for their advice. In particular, the Alzheimer's Society's publications have been an invaluable source of clear and accurate information. A number of colleagues have read and commented on the text as we have gone along. Responsibility for the content of the book is, however, ours and ours alone.

We extend special thanks to the following people with dementia who read the previous edition and made many helpful suggestions:

Christine Bryden
Alzheimer's Society: The Living with Dementia team and
    working group
The Forget Me Not Centre, Swindon

We also thank:
Janet Baylis, Manager, Dementia Knowledge Centre, Alzheimer's
    Society
Helen Krizka and members of the Camden Carer support group of
    the Alzheimer's Society for providing many of the questions.

Steve Milton from Innovations in Dementia, Rachel Canning and Frederika Stradling read and commented on the manuscript for this third edition. Our thanks go to all three of them.

Introduction

If you are a person affected by dementia, this book is for you. You may have recently been told your diagnosis, you may be caring for someone with memory loss, you may know someone who has dementia. Whoever you are, the confusion that is the main feature of dementia does not affect only the person with the condition. Carers, family members and friends are also bewildered and confused by what is happening to the person they know. Often when the diagnosis is first made you do not think of all the questions that you want to ask or you may feel you are not ready to ask them. But as time passes you will probably want to know as much as possible about dementia and how to care for someone who has it. Knowledge is the best way of lifting the cloud of confusion and taking charge of the situation for yourself.

Although this book is written mainly for people with dementia and their family and carers, it will also be useful for care workers in the community and in hospitals and residential and nursing homes. Many of the questions answered, particularly about communication, behaviour and treatments, are the same whoever you are or wherever you are working. People who have been given a diagnosis of dementia may find parts of the book useful, perhaps particularly those on dementia itself and on legal and financial arrangements. As earlier diagnosis is achieved, more people with dementia want and are able to plan their own treatment and care.

This book is about all types of dementia, including Alzheimer's disease, which is the most common type, and vascular dementia, which is second most common. Although members of the public quite often use the name Alzheimer's disease to refer to dementia in general, in this book the name is used only for that particular type of dementia. Most of the questions and answers will be relevant whatever form of dementia you are concerned with.

The book answers 276 questions. All of them are real questions asked by carers, by friends and family members and by people with dementia themselves. We have tried to answer them as clearly and as accurately as we can. Research into Alzheimer's disease and other dementias is moving fast, new treatments are becoming available and, of course, the law on mental health and on benefits is subject to change, so you will need to check on the details if you are using this book some time after it was published.

You will probably not want to read this book from cover to cover. Some chapters will be relevant to you at different stages of the condition. The usefulness of some parts will depend on the type of dementia that concerns you, or on your financial circumstances, or on your relationship to the person you care for. This is a book to refer to as and when you need to. We hope it will be easy to dip into. Each question and answer is self-contained and there are cross-references to other questions and answers whenever that seems helpful.

The first chapter of the book answers questions about the different types and causes of dementia. Chapter 2 is concerned specifically with Alzheimer's disease. Chapters 3 to 8 aim to help you with the practical issues of looking after someone with dementia. In Chapter 9 we explain where you can get help and in Chapter 11 the financial and legal arrangements that can be made to assist you. Chapter 10 looks at care in residential and nursing homes. Chapter 12 describes different types of treatment and the final chapter looks at current and future research.

No one book on dementia is ever going to be enough. We have added a reading list of other publications that we hope will be helpful to you. There is also an appendix giving the names, addresses and websites of some useful organisations. These will be valuable sources of up-to-date information.

It isn't easy being someone with dementia or caring for them but, as we hope this book shows, many difficulties can be overcome. Sharing your problems and feelings with others is perhaps the most important thing you can do. Organisations such as the Alzheimer's

Society, Alzheimer Scotland and the Alzheimer Society of Ireland are there with information, practical help and emotional support.

This book was first published in 1997 under the title of *Alzheimer's at your fingertips*. This third edition, with its new title of *Alzheimer's and other Dementias*, includes comprehensively updated information on medical, social, legal and financial developments concerning people with dementia and those who care for them.

We, the authors, thank all the readers who wrote to us after reading the earlier editions of the book. We value your comments and ask readers once again to let us know if you would like to add to any of our answers or if you think we could offer other useful advice. We would also like to know if there are important questions that we have not included. Please write to us c/o Class Publishing, Barb House, Barb Mews, London W6 7PA, UK.

1 | What is dementia?

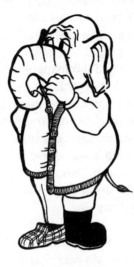

There are many different types of dementia. This chapter will give you information on what dementia is and on most types of dementia other than Alzheimer's disease. Because Alzheimer's disease is the most common type, we describe it separately in Chapter 2. In all types there is a decline in mental function, especially memory, and disturbance of daily activities and social relationships.

DEFINING DEMENTIA

What is dementia?

'Dementia' is a term used to describe various different brain disorders that have in common loss of brain function, which is usually progressive and eventually severe. There are over 100 different types of dementia. The most common are Alzheimer's disease, vascular dementia and Lewy body dementia.

People with dementia have particular problems with their short-term memory. They consistently forget things that they have just said or done, even though they can often recall clearly events that happened many years ago. Their sense of time and place is typically lost as the disease progresses. They may develop problems with finding words, and it becomes increasingly difficult for them to learn new information and to do new things. As time goes on, people with dementia need help to do even the most basic tasks of everyday living, including washing, dressing and eating. Eventually, people with dementia may become uncommunicative and incontinent. Sometimes there are severe behavioural problems. Most people with dementia eventually require 24-hour care. Whatever the type of dementia (see below), the disease often goes on for many years, and often people die of something else.

My family tell me that my grandmother became 'senile' before she died. Does this mean she had senile dementia or could she have had Alzheimer's disease?

People quite often use the term 'senile' to describe old people who have become confused in their thoughts. Strictly speaking, the word 'senile' just means old, but people have often used it in common speech to mean senile dementia (an unhelpful term that should not be used).

If your grandmother's 'senility' lasted for months or years before she died, it is likely that she did have some form of dementia, and the most common form of dementia is Alzheimer's disease (see Chapter 2). However, if your grandmother's mental problems developed only in the last weeks or months of her life, it is more likely that she did not have dementia but that her brain function was being affected by a disease elsewhere in her body, such as the liver, kidneys or heart.

As people get older they tend to become more forgetful, but this is sometimes part of the natural ageing process rather than dementia.

(See the section 'Symptoms and signs' in Chapter 2 for information on how Alzheimer's disease and other dementias differ from ordinary forgetfulness.) Some people refer to any older person who is a bit forgetful as being senile, but this term should not be used at all.

I'm 52 and have been told I have early-onset Alzheimer's disease. What is this? Is it the same as 'pre-senile dementia'?

Although the term pre-senile dementia sometimes still appears in textbooks, it should not be used. In the past, the distinction tended to be made around the age of 60. 'Senile dementia' is just another term for dementia appearing in older people. Most of what used to be called pre-senile dementia and senile dementia are in fact Alzheimer's disease.

At 52 you are quite young to be diagnosed with dementia. In fact, fewer than 2 in 100 cases of dementia occur in people under 65, so it is quite possible that, in the past, your dementia would have been referred to as 'pre-senile'. Having dementia so young can bring its own set of problems because people may still be at work and have young children. Another problem is that many areas of the UK do not have specific services for younger people with dementia. Although Alzheimer's is the most common cause of dementia in people under 65, there are many other uncommon causes which may require specialist assessment. For this reason, it may be best for you to have an opinion from a neurologist or psychiatrist specialising in this field.

I have been told that my next-door neighbour has dementia but that she does not have Alzheimer's disease. What other sorts of dementia are there?

There are a number of different types of dementia. All of these affect the brain and cause a progressive loss of memory that may eventually make it impossible for the affected person to perform even the simplest everyday tasks without help.

Alzheimer's disease (see Chapter 2) is the most common type of dementia, accounting on its own for about half of all cases. There are, however, quite a number of other types of dementia and it seems that your neighbour has been diagnosed with one of these. Among these other types of dementia, all but vascular and Lewy body dementia are rare.

Types of dementia other than Alzheimer's disease include:

- vascular dementia, which is usually the result of brain damage due to tiny strokes;

- Lewy body dementia, which has some features in common with Parkinson's disease;

- fronto-temporal dementia, for example Pick's disease, in which there are striking changes in behaviour before the memory problems appear;

- Huntington's disease, also sometimes called Huntington's chorea, which is characterised by jerky movements in addition to dementia;

- AIDS-related dementia;

- dementia that sometimes occurs together with Parkinson's disease;

- Creutzfeldt–Jakob disease (CJD);

- dementia due to a brain tumour;

- normal pressure hydrocephalus, due to a build-up of fluid in the brain;

- dementia due to an excessive intake of alcohol over an extended period of time;

- dementias due to various treatable causes, including vitamin deficiency, hormone deficiency and syphilis.

These different types are discussed later in this chapter.

WHO WILL GET DEMENTIA?

How common is dementia, and is it more common in some groups of people than others?

The chances of developing some form of dementia increase with age, but dementia does occur very rarely in people under the age of 60. Over the age of 65, dementia affects approximately 6 people in 100. For people over 80, the number affected rises to 20 in 100. Similar rates are seen in other countries across Europe. It is estimated that there are currently about 700,000 people with dementia in the UK, and this is set to double by 2050. Some researchers have suggested that there are over 24 million people world-wide who have dementia, with 4.6 million new cases annually.

In general, dementia seems to affect all groups in society equally. It is not known to be particularly linked with gender, social class, ethnic group or geographic location.

CAUSES OF DEMENTIA

Can stress or worry cause dementia?

There is no evidence that stress or worry is responsible for causing dementia. However, stress or worry can lead to forgetfulness and confusion that may sometimes be mistaken for early dementia. It is also true that a diagnosis of dementia is sometimes made only after a period of stress or worry has made the disease more apparent, even though the dementia has in fact been present for some time. Anxiety is a common symptom of depression in older people and the presence of depression can result in severe memory problems that may be mistaken for dementia.

My husband has been told that he has some sort of dementia and that he should give up smoking. Can smoking cause dementia?

Smoking is not thought to be a direct cause of dementia, but it can contribute to heart disease and atherosclerosis (narrowing of the arteries), which often leads to strokes. One form of dementia, called vascular dementia, is often caused by strokes, which cause brain damage by cutting off the blood supply to areas of the brain.

Not all doctors agree that giving up smoking is likely to have much effect on the course of dementia once this disease is already apparent, and you may find that your husband has difficulty stopping smoking. However, stopping smoking can be recommended on many other health grounds, and *may* help to prevent strokes which could make his dementia worse. A lot of help is now available for people who want to stop smoking. Your husband's GP will be able to help or you could phone Quit – a charity dedicated to help people stop smoking – for advice (contact details in Appendix 1).

My father, who is 72, has recently had an operation on his bowel. He was a bit forgetful before he went into hospital but now he is home again he is very confused. Might the operation have given him dementia?

Some older people have temporary confusion after an operation. The after-effects of the anaesthetic and taking pain-relieving drugs may increase confusion for a short time. Confusion may also be made worse by having to cope with the unfamiliar environment of the hospital.

If your father's confusion persists, it is possible that he did have dementia before the operation, which has been made worse. Occasionally, dementia can be triggered by an operation: during an operation older people may be vulnerable to having little strokes or temporary problems with the blood supply to the brain, which can cause lasting confusion.

Another possible explanation for your father's increased confusion is that he has picked up a chest or urinary tract infection. This possibility is less likely if the operation was some time ago. However, do speak to his doctor about your concerns, as treatment of an infection or a change in your husband's medication can sometimes bring about a dramatic improvement.

Can head injuries cause dementia?

People who suffer severe or repeated head injuries may be at increased risk of developing dementia. However, the link between head injuries and dementia is not straightforward. It is possible that a head injury may trigger the disease process in susceptible individuals. People who have sustained serious head injuries through boxing are prone to a type of dementia known as 'dementia pugilistica', which is similar to Alzheimer's disease.

TYPES OF DEMENTIA

What are the types of dementia?

There are many different types of dementia, with different possible causes. In many cases, the types are not fully understood. For example, dementia in general is much more common in older people, but the ageing process as such is not considered to be an actual cause of dementia.

A few types of dementia, such as Pick's disease and Huntington's disease (see later in this section) and rare cases of Alzheimer's disease (see Chapter 2), are known to be inherited, passed on from one generation to the next in the genes. Other types of dementia, including most cases of Alzheimer's disease and also vascular dementia, are thought to be caused by a combination of genetic and other factors.

Some types of dementia occur as a feature of some other disease, such as AIDS, Parkinson's disease and syphilis.

A person's behaviour can also increase the risk of dementia, even if it does not directly cause it. People who smoke, for example, have an increased risk for vascular dementia and people whose alcohol consumption is excessive may develop alcoholic dementia or Korsakoff's syndrome.

What is vascular dementia?

Vascular dementia (also known as multi-infarct dementia) is caused by insufficient blood supply to the brain. It is the second most common type of dementia in the UK, after Alzheimer's disease. Vascular dementia is estimated to account on its own for about one in five dementia cases, and to occur with Alzheimer's disease in another one in five cases.

There are various causes of vascular dementia, the most common probably being a series of 'mini strokes' (known as infarcts). A stroke destroys an area of cells in the brain by cutting off the blood supply. A stroke can be so slight that it causes no immediate symptoms, or may just cause a brief spell of dizziness, weakness or confusion. Eventually this damage accumulates sufficiently to cause dementia.

Strokes may occur because of high blood pressure, which can cause blood vessels in the brain to burst, or because of blood clots, which can cause blockages in the vessels supplying blood to the brain. People who smoke, have high blood pressure or diabetes or are overweight seem to be at increased risk of strokes.

Even though the damage caused by an individual stroke may be slight, the cumulative effect is often sufficient to cause dementia. Sometimes people can get dementia after a single stroke if it affects a crucial part of the brain. Some people develop dementia because the blood supply to the whole brain is reduced for a short period of time; for example, because of a heart attack or during an operation. The brain only needs to have a poor blood supply for one or two minutes for lasting damage to result.

The main symptoms of vascular dementia, like most other dementias, are loss of short-term memory, loss of sense of time and a progressive decline in other abilities. However, in vascular dementia, the memory loss is typically much more variable than in Alzheimer's disease, and people with this type of dementia can be much better some days than others. There may be long periods when a person's memory loss does not seem to get worse, and can even improve; and then there may be an episode of acute confusion (often associated with a new mini stroke) followed by a step down in the person's memory. Doctors describe vascular dementia as having a 'step-like' progression.

Other characteristic features of vascular dementia are that people usually have a greater degree of awareness of their disability than is the case in Alzheimer's disease. There may be a relative preservation of personality but an increased likelihood of problems with unpredictable behaviour or changeable emotions.

My father never used to use bad language and now he swears all the time. I've been told he has 'frontal lobe symptoms'. What does this mean?

'Frontal lobe' refers to the front areas of the brain, just behind the eyes. If the frontal lobes stop working properly, different symptoms can emerge:

- Change in personality; people can become more placid or, occasionally, more aggressive or irritable.

- Loss of motivation.

- People just lose their 'get up and go' and become more uninterested in things. This may also happen in depression, Parkinson's disease and other conditions.

- Loss of the ability to plan and organise.

- Loss of restraint – the technical term for this is 'disinhibition'.

- People may swear, say rude things, laugh inappropriately or become sexually disinhibited.

There is no fixed pattern of symptoms. People with this condition may have any combination of the typical symptoms, and these may change over time. Eventually, any type of dementia can cause frontal lobe symptoms but some types of dementia (for example, Pick's disease – see the next answer) begin with frontal symptoms.

It seems that my mother has a type of dementia called fronto-temporal dementia. What is this? How does it differ from Alzheimer's disease?

Fronto-temporal dementia (one type of which is called Pick's disease, after the doctor who first described it) is a rare type of dementia. It has various similarities with Alzheimer's disease (see Chapter 2), but also differs from that disease in a number of important respects.

Fronto-temporal dementia typically develops at an earlier age than Alzheimer's disease, usually in a person's 40s or 50s. It is thought to have a genetic cause in some families, but it can also occur when there is no family history of this form of dementia.

The most important difference between fronto-temporal dementia and Alzheimer's disease is that the brain tissue changes that occur in fronto-temporal dementia typically affect mainly the frontal lobes of the brain. It causes marked shrinkage of these lobes while leaving other parts of the brain relatively unaffected.

As with Alzheimer's disease, a definite diagnosis of fronto-temporal dementia disease requires a post-mortem examination (autopsy). However, in practice, the diagnosis can often be made from a person's symptoms and signs. If a doctor suspects fronto-temporal dementia, he or she will sometimes ask a psychologist to do specific tests that can help the diagnosis.

Many of the early symptoms of fronto-temporal dementia are 'frontal lobe symptoms' (see the previous answer). These can be very subtle in the early stages of the illness, and it may take many months, or even years, for anyone, including doctors, to suspect that the person has dementia.

Another feature of fronto-temporal dementia is that some people with this condition may start by having problems with language. This is because the area of the brain that is involved in creating speech is in the frontal lobe. It may seem like the person can't find the right words, or no longer understands words that were previously familiar to them (known as 'semantic dementia') or some people may progressively lose their speech altogether (known as 'primary progressive aphasia').

The outlook for people with fronto-temporal dementia is similar to that for people with Alzheimer's disease. A progressive decline in abilities will typically lead to death between five and ten years after diagnosis.

My boyfriend says he doesn't want to get serious with me because there is Huntington's disease in his family. What does this mean?

Huntington's disease is a relatively rare form of dementia in which mental deterioration is accompanied by problems in controlling body movements. Huntington's disease is an inherited disease. If your boyfriend's mother or father has the disease, there is a one in two chance that he (and also any of his brothers or sisters) will also develop it.

People at risk of developing Huntington's disease can have genetic counselling and then a genetic test to find out whether or not they have inherited the abnormal gene that will give them the disease. However, it is important to respect a person's wishes if he or she prefers not to find out this information in advance.

Huntington's disease usually becomes apparent when someone who has inherited the disease reaches his or her 30s or 40s, although symptoms can start sooner. The illness may begin with either mental or physical symptoms. Progressive loss of memory and concentration, leading to severe dementia, may be accompanied by anxiety, irritability and depression. The movement problems that characterise this disease take the form of involuntary twitching and

spasms of the muscles. There is no specific treatment for Huntington's disease, but drugs do sometimes help the movement problems.
The illness typically lasts for 10 to 25 years, leading to severe disability. As the disease progresses, 24-hour nursing care will inevitably
be needed.

Do most people with HIV develop dementia?

Most people infected with HIV – the virus that leads to AIDS – do
not develop dementia. However, there is a possibility that
someone with HIV may develop subtle memory problems before
developing AIDS.

Some people (probably less than 5%) who have AIDS develop
severe dementia, which is often characterised by apathy and problems with clumsiness and walking. In some people with AIDS, the
dementia that accompanies it is due to a direct effect of the HIV virus
on the brain. In others, the dementia is due to an infection or a
tumour of the brain that develops because of lowered immunity due
to HIV.

There are now treatments – called anti-retroviral therapy – for
people with AIDS, which may help to reverse some of the symptoms
of dementia. The treatment can be complicated and involves several
tablets taken at different times of the day. For this reason it is better
to make sure that people who have memory problems associated
with AIDS always have their treatments supervised.

My father has had Parkinson's disease for three years now and seems to be getting quite forgetful. I have heard that people with Parkinson's sometimes develop dementia – is this true?

It is true that people with Parkinson's disease do have an increased
risk of developing dementia, usually starting at least two years
after the Parkinson's disease begins. This is known as 'Parkinson's
disease dementia' and affects an estimated 15–20% of people with
Parkinson's disease. However, the fact that your father is showing

signs of forgetfulness does not necessarily mean that he is developing dementia. It is possible that your father's memory is working perfectly well and that he only appears to have a memory problem because he is slowed down by the Parkinson's disease.

Even if he does have a memory problem, this may not be due to dementia. For example, people who have Parkinson's disease are often treated with drugs belonging to a drug group known as anticholinergics (see Glossary). These drugs can reduce the symptoms of Parkinson's disease but they also sometimes make someone's memory worse. Also, people who have Parkinson's disease sometimes become depressed. Depression is a common cause of poor memory, which is sometimes misinterpreted as dementia (see Chapter 3 for more information on depression and dementia).

Some people develop symptoms of Parkinson's disease at around the same time as they show signs of dementia. If this happens, they are more likely to have Lewy body dementia (see the next answer for more information).

I thought my husband had Alzheimer's disease but the specialist says that it is Lewy body dementia. What are the differences? Will the fact that my husband has Lewy body dementia affect how I can look after him?

Lewy body dementia is a form of dementia that is similar to Alzheimer's disease. It takes its name from abnormal collections of protein, known as Lewy bodies, that occur in the nerve cells of the brain.

Your husband probably has symptoms and signs similar to those of someone with Parkinson's disease, such as having a tremor, being somewhat unsteady on his feet and being rather slowed down. He may also be experiencing visual hallucinations (see the section 'Hallucinations' in Chapter 7) and may have started to have falls. Some people with Lewy body dementia have more confusion at night. It is also likely that your husband's condition will vary from day to day, and that on some days he will have a short episode of being very confused, which will then settle. This pattern is typical of Lewy body dementia but is not common in Alzheimer's disease.

In terms of care, your husband's needs will be much the same as if he had been found to have Alzheimer's disease rather than Lewy body dementia. The main difference is that you may find it more difficult to predict how he is going to feel on a day-to-day basis compared with someone with Alzheimer's disease.

People with Lewy body dementia are very sensitive to tranquillisers known as antipsychotic or neuroleptic drugs, and for this reason use of these drugs should be avoided if at all possible.

My wife, who is 75, started to lose her memory about ten years ago and five years ago was diagnosed with Alzheimer's disease. We have both eaten a lot of beef. Do you think she might have CJD not Alzheimer's?

Your wife is very unlikely to have CJD (Creutzfeldt–Jakob disease). CJD is an extremely rare type of dementia that affects only one in a million people in the UK, whereas Alzheimer's disease (see Chapter 2) affects around one in ten people of your wife's age. However, the main reason for thinking that your wife is unlikely to have CJD is that her illness has now lasted for a number of years. CJD usually progresses very rapidly and is usually fatal within a year.

Many of the early signs of CJD are similar to Alzheimer's disease but there are some differences. People with CJD may become rather withdrawn and forgetful, and soon develop problems in finding the right words and having a conversation. They also become unsteady on their feet and frequently have spasms or jerky movements in their arms and legs.

Over the last few years, there has been a lot of publicity about a link between CJD and BSE (bovine spongiform encephalopathy), a similar disease that affects cows. CJD, BSE and a disease called scrapie (in sheep) are all known to be caused by an unusual infectious particle called a prion. In recent years a number of cases of CJD have occurred in mainly younger people. These cases are thought to be linked to eating beef from cows infected with BSE. Their illness is now considered to be a distinctive new form of CJD known as variant CJD (vCJD). No link has been found between beef eating and the more usual forms of CJD, which typically develops in old age. (More information is available from the CJD Support Network and the Human BSE Foundation campaigns for families affected by vCJD; see Appendix 1 for contact details.)

Might dementia be due to a brain tumour?

Brain tumours are a rare cause of dementia. One type of slow-growing brain tumour, known as a meningioma, sometimes causes symptoms of dementia. Most brain tumours cause other kinds of symptoms, such as loss of limb function, visual disturbance and loss of balance. In some cases, removal of a meningioma may result in recovery from the dementia.

Can 'water on the brain' cause dementia?

The rare type of dementia known as 'normal pressure hydrocephalus' is due not to water but to an excess of cerebrospinal fluid in the brain.

Early symptoms of this type of dementia include incontinence of urine and problems with walking. If your doctor suspects this type of dementia, he or she may order a brain scan to confirm the diagnosis. This type of dementia may be helped by an operation (see the section 'Surgery' in Chapter 12).

Can hormone deficiencies cause dementia?

Under-activity of the thyroid gland (a gland in the neck that regulates our metabolism) can result in a condition called 'hypothyroidism', of which dementia can be a symptom. People with hypothyroidism typically gain weight and develop a hoarse voice, dry skin and thinning hair. Hypothyroidism can be simply treated with replacement thyroid hormones. Some other hormone deficiencies are rare causes of dementia.

Does drinking too much alcohol cause dementia?

People who drink too much alcohol over a prolonged period of time may develop dementia in addition to many other health problems.

Some heavy drinkers have a specific problem of loss of short-term memory, known as Korsakoff's syndrome, which develops because of vitamin B_1 (thiamine) deficiency. This results in difficulty in learning new information, although old memories and other aspects of brain function are often preserved. Others develop a wider range of problems that resemble Alzheimer's disease. Drinking moderate amounts of alcohol is probably safe, and some researchers have suggested that small amounts of alcohol (about 1 glass of wine per day or equivalent) may actually reduce the chance of developing dementia.

Can dietary deficiencies cause dementia? My wife has been a vegetarian for many years and now has dementia. Could her diet be to blame?

It is true that dietary deficiencies are a rare cause of dementia. However, it is very unlikely that your wife's dementia has been caused by her vegetarianism. Your wife is much more likely to have one of the more common types of dementia, such as Alzheimer's disease.

Deficiencies of some vitamins, such as vitamin B_{12} or B_1 (thiamine), have been suggested as rare causes of dementia. These vitamins are present in a wide range of foods and can be stored by the body for long periods. However, it is uncommon for anyone to develop a deficiency of either of these vitamins.

People who drink excessive amounts of alcohol over a long period of time sometimes develop a deficiency of vitamin B_1, leading to a condition called Korsakoff 's syndrome (discussed in the previous answer). People on a vegan diet, which excludes not only meat but also eggs and milk, may need supplementary vitamin B_{12}.

A few people develop a deficiency of vitamin B_{12} because their bodies do not absorb this vitamin properly. This is usually because of a condition called 'pernicious anaemia' – due either to a rare stomach problem, known as 'intrinsic factor deficiency', or to previous surgery to the bowel.

Although dementia due to vitamin deficiency is rare, your wife's doctor will probably have already carried out a blood test to exclude this possibility. In cases where a vitamin B_{12} deficiency is found, the usual treatment is to give the vitamin by injection every three months.

2 | What is Alzheimer's disease?

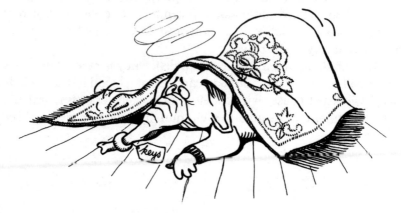

Alzheimer's disease is the most common type of dementia. This chapter tells you about Alzheimer's disease, what we know about its causes, how it damages the brain and its effect on people who have it. Although there are many similarities between different types of dementia, it helps to distinguish between them and to understand the differences. The more we know about Alzheimer's disease, the better care we can give.

DEFINING ALZHEIMER'S DISEASE

Where did Alzheimer's disease get its name?

Alzheimer's disease is named after Dr Alois Alzheimer, a German neurologist (1864–1915), who in 1906 observed changes in the brain tissue of a woman in her 50s, called Auguste D, who had died of what was thought to be an unusual mental illness. These abnormal brain tissue changes are now known to be the characteristic features of Alzheimer's disease.

The term 'dementia' sometimes seems to be used instead of 'Alzheimer's disease'. Are they two names for the same thing?

Dementia is a term used to describe various disorders of the brain that usually result in progressive and severe loss of memory. Alzheimer's disease is one type of dementia. There are many others and the common ones are discussed in this book. Alzheimer's disease is the most common dementia, accounting on its own for roughly 50% of all cases (and occurring with another cause in a further 20% of cases).

What happens when someone develops Alzheimer's disease?

People with Alzheimer's disease (and other dementias) gradually lose their sense of time and place. A major symptom is that they forget things that they have just said or done, although their memory for past events may remain clear for a time. As the disease progresses, people become unaware of their condition although they may still experience distress. They find it increasingly difficult and then impossible to perform even the simplest everyday tasks – including washing, eating and dressing – without supervision. They may become uncommunicative and incontinent, sometimes with severe behavioural problems. Many eventually need 24-hour care.

The disease may go on for many years – typically between five and ten years – and tends not to be the eventual cause of death. More commonly, a person has Alzheimer's disease for many years before dying from something else, such as an infection or a stroke. See other questions in this book for more information about the different types of dementia.

Has everyone with memory loss got Alzheimer's disease or some other kind of dementia?

No. There are many other causes of memory problems. As people get older, many are aware that their memory is not as good as it used to be. Often this is just a part of normal ageing and is not dementia (see also the section 'Symptoms and signs' later in this chapter).

Other conditions that cause symptoms that may be mistaken for dementia include deafness and depression, and short periods of confusion may occur for other reasons, such as chest infections, heart problems, and sometimes after surgery. Some medicines can make some older people confused. For these reasons it is a good idea for everybody who has problems with their memory to be seen by a doctor.

Is it true that the only certain way of knowing if someone has had Alzheimer's disease is to carry out a post-mortem examination of the brain?

In most cases, an absolutely certain diagnosis of Alzheimer's disease usually depends on finding characteristic changes in the brain tissue. These changes can be found only during the course of a post-mortem examination (an autopsy), so it's not possible until the person has died. Spread throughout the brains of people who have died of Alzheimer's disease are deposits, or 'plaques', made up of an abnormal protein called beta-amyloid. A further abnormality is the occurrence of tangles of twisted protein molecules within the nerve cells of the brain. Other features – also found in other dementias – are shrinkage of the brain and widespread death of nerve cells.

In rare cases, where a person has a gene that is known to cause an inherited form of Alzheimer's disease (see the section 'Who will get Alzheimer's disease?' below), a test for that gene can confirm the diagnosis.

However, in practice, the diagnosis of Alzheimer's disease is usually made on the basis of identifying that a person has symptoms of some form of dementia, and then ruling out various conditions other than Alzheimer's disease that might be the cause. (See Chapter 3 for more about diagnosis.) After a full assessment of the patient, doctors can usually tell whether someone has Alzheimer's disease or another type of dementia or is not suffering from dementia at all, without examining brain tissue.

What is the difference between senile dementia and Alzheimer's disease?

The term 'senile dementia' was formerly used when people 'lost their memory' at an older age. This loss of memory was thought to be part of the normal ageing process. However, it is now appreciated that most people do not develop dementia even at a great age. Most of what used to be called senile dementia was in fact Alzheimer's disease or another dementia.

Alzheimer's disease is the same disease at whatever age it occurs. In the past, however, a distinction used to be made on the basis of age. Older people were described as having senile dementia, while younger ones were said to have pre-senile dementia. This distinction is now widely considered unhelpful and misleading and the term 'senile' (which means 'old') should not be used.

WHO WILL GET ALZHEIMER'S DISEASE?

A lot of people now seem to be developing Alzheimer's disease. How common is it? And is it on the increase?

Alzheimer's disease is very rare in younger people but becomes more common with increasing age. It can affect people as young as 30, but this is very rare. Up to the age of 65, Alzheimer's disease develops in only about 1 person in 1,000. In older people, the disease becomes more common, affecting around 3 people in 100 over the age of 65. Over the age of 80, this figure rises to between 10 and 15 per 100.

The number of people who currently have Alzheimer's disease in the UK is approaching 400,000 (and a further 300,000 have other forms of dementia). These numbers are increasing. This increase is due partly to earlier and better diagnosis but mainly to the fact that more people are now living longer and reaching an age at which the risk of developing Alzheimer's disease is increased.

Does Alzheimer's disease run in families?

Alzheimer's disease does sometimes run in families, but this is very uncommon. Some rare cases of the disease, which tend to occur in younger people than usual, are known to be inherited and are passed on by a single gene from one generation to the next. (For more information on the inherited form of Alzheimer's disease, see the next answer, and also the second answer in the section 'Causes of Alzheimer's disease', below.) In these very rare cases, the probability that close family members (brothers, sisters and children) will develop Alzheimer's disease is one in two.

The vast majority of cases of Alzheimer's disease are not of the type that is passed on by a single gene. In this *non-genetic* form of the disease, the risk to close relatives is a little higher than in a person of a similar age who has no family history of Alzheimer's. For example, someone at the age of 70 with no family history has about a 1 in 50 chance of developing Alzheimer's disease during their 70th year. This would increase to about a 1 in 20 chance in someone with a close relative who had Alzheimer's.

How would I know if my family has the inherited form of Alzheimer's disease? And how likely would this make me to get the disease?

The form of Alzheimer's disease that is definitely known to be passed on from one generation to the next in the genes is extremely rare. It is very unlikely that your family has it unless close relatives have developed the disease under the age of 60. Characteristics of this inherited form of Alzheimer's disease are that it develops at a younger age than usual, typically between the ages of 35 and 60, and that it tends to develop at a similar age within the family.

If your family does have this inherited form of Alzheimer's disease, you are at risk only if your mother or father developed it. If one of them did develop it, you have a one in two chance of developing the disease. In these circumstances, a genetic test (see the section 'Genetic tests' later in this chapter) could be requested to confirm whether or not you do in fact have the gene for this disease.

CAUSES OF ALZHEIMER'S DISEASE

How much is known about the possible causes of Alzheimer's disease?

This is an important area of current research, but at the present time a great deal still remains to be discovered about why people develop Alzheimer's disease.

We know that Alzheimer's disease becomes more common with increasing age, but we don't know what factors trigger the characteristic changes that occur in the brain tissue of people who have this disease. We do know, however, that these brain changes are not part of the normal ageing process – in some cases, the changes occur at a relatively early age.

Genes are thought to play a part in the development of most cases of Alzheimer's disease. In very rare cases, abnormal genes actually cause the disease (see the previous answer). Much more commonly, genes are believed only to contribute to a person's susceptibility to the disease.

Alzheimer's disease is certainly not infectious. Even though the disease is sometimes first noticed after a period of stress or worry, it is not thought that these emotions can actually cause the disease to develop. Claims are sometimes made that dietary or hormone deficiencies may contribute to the development of Alzheimer's disease. Most doctors do not accept these claims. Similarly, claims that aluminium in the diet may be a cause (discussed later in this section) are not widely accepted.

Some things have been shown to be linked with an increased risk of developing Alzheimer's disease. These include high blood pressure, having too much cholesterol in the blood and being very overweight. It is possible that head injury in earlier life may increase the chance of developing Alzheimer's disease in later life.

How do genes cause Alzheimer's disease?

Research suggests that the genes associated with the development of Alzheimer's disease might have an effect on chemicals known as *neurotransmitters*, which allow messages to be communicated between nerve cells. One type of neurotransmitter, called acetylcholine, is known to be deficient in people with Alzheimer's disease.

Another way in which abnormal genes might exert their effect is through their influence on nerve growth factor (a chemical in the brain that stimulates the growth and development of nerve cells). It is thought that genes might interfere with the way that this factor normally enhances the growth of functioning nerve cells to compensate for the death of other cells.

Recently, research has focused on a gene that makes a protein called *apolipoprotein E* (ApoE). All people carry two of these Apo-E genes, which help to regulate cholesterol in the blood. There are three types of ApoE – e2, e3 and e4. Each person inherits an ApoE gene from each parent. It seems that people who carry two ApoE-e4 genes (one from each parent) have a higher risk of developing Alzheimer's disease.

Abnormalities on three other genes – PS1 (presenilin type 1), PS2 (presenilin type 2) and APP (amyloid precursor protein) – have been identified as causes of the rare inherited form of the disease, but it is not clear how they do this.

Why do people with Down's syndrome develop Alzheimer's disease?

People with Down's syndrome nearly always have an extra chromosome 21. One gene on chromosome 21 codes for or creates amyloid precursor protein (APP). Abnormal amounts of amyloid in the brain occur in Alzheimer's disease. It seems that the extra gene results in an excess of amyloid. Consequently, it is thought that over 50% of people with Down's syndrome over the age of 40 have Alzheimer's disease

Does aluminium cause Alzheimer's disease? Is it safe to use aluminium saucepans?

A number of research findings have suggested a possible link between aluminium and Alzheimer's disease. These findings include: the presence of aluminium deposits in tangles and plaques (discussed in the section 'Defining Alzheimer's disease' earlier) in the brains of people with Alzheimer's disease; and increased rates of dementia in people with kidney failure whose bodies have raised levels of aluminium. However, a large study of the brains of people who had died from Alzheimer's disease found only normal levels of aluminium.

Some studies have suggested that people living in areas with high concentrations of aluminium in the water supply may be more likely to develop Alzheimer's disease. However, this evidence is inconclusive. Exposure to aluminium from other sources, such as from drinking tea, using antiperspirants and taking antacids, has not been shown to be linked to the development of Alzheimer's disease.

Because there is only weak or circumstantial evidence for linking aluminium with the development of Alzheimer's disease, there seems to be little justification for not using aluminium cooking utensils.

Might mercury in dental fillings cause Alzheimer's?

This is not thought to be likely. Mercury has been shown to be toxic to the central nervous system, but this does not prove any link with Alzheimer's disease. Nor is a link proved by unconfirmed research suggesting that the brains of people with Alzheimer's disease might contain more mercury than normal.

What can I do to stop myself getting Alzheimer's disease? If I keep my brain active, will this help?

The simple answer to this is nobody knows for certain. Some research recently has shown that people who are more intelligent than others may be less likely to develop dementia, and Alzheimer's disease in particular, in later life. However, the reasons for this are not clear. One possible explanation is that the more we use our brains, the more able our brains are to cope with the effects of dementia. So, the best advice is that it is probably good to keep your brain active.

It is increasingly thought that Alzheimer's disease may be linked with vascular disease (discussed in the section 'Types of dementia' in Chapter 1), high blood pressure and being overweight, so a healthy lifestyle, with good food and regular exercise, and not smoking, may be helpful. Some researchers have suggested that drinking moderate amounts of alcohol (for example, one glass of wine) every day may reduce the chance of developing Alzheimer's.

Currently, scientists are looking at whether substances such as vitamin E, oestrogen and other chemicals may prevent dementia, but this seems unlikely.

SYMPTOMS AND SIGNS

I am really worried. My husband had Alzheimer's disease and now I am beginning to forget things as well. Am I developing dementia?

This is a very common worry. As people get older they find that their memory is not as good as it used to be and many people worry that they are developing dementia, especially if they have had a family member with the illness. This is not necessarily the case. For example, as people get older they have more difficulty in remembering people's names or things they are going to buy in the shop. They may also forget appointments. If you are doing this, it does not mean that you are getting Alzheimer's disease.

Someone with ordinary forgetfulness can still remember the details associated with the thing they have forgotten. For example, you may briefly forget your next-door neighbour's name but you still know that the person you are talking to is the next-door neighbour. People with dementia forget not only the details but the entire context as well. People with dementia usually also have other problems, such as changes in behaviour or personality, and they may lose the ability to perform everyday tasks or have problems with their speech.

There are other possible reasons why your memory may not be as good as it used to be. For example, you may be getting depressed or suffering from stress. For this reason, if you are concerned about your memory, it may be worthwhile visiting your doctor to have a check-up.

What are the tell-tale signs of the onset of Alzheimer's disease? What should I be looking out for?

One of the changes that often appear when someone is in the early stages of Alzheimer's disease is that the person seems different from their usual self, but in ways that are hard to pinpoint.

The person may seem less capable, less involved and less adaptable. You may notice that they lose interest in hobbies and pastimes. They may show loss of concentration, may be unable to make decisions and seem to avoid taking responsibility. They may also show some odd behaviours, such as getting ready to go to work many years after they have retired. The person may be showing odd mood changes, such as irritability and suspicion, which may be due to becoming aware that something is wrong but not knowing quite what the problem is. A common early problem is very mild memory difficulties, such as forgetting appointments or losing track of conversations; but these are also frequent in people who are not developing dementia.

All these changes occur very gradually with Alzheimer's and are quite difficult to pick up early on. They are more often identified when looking back and trying to work out what the first signs of the disease were.

Does Alzheimer's disease differ from one person to another?

Alzheimer's disease does affect people differently. Although the disease tends to follow a broadly similar pattern – a progressive decline in mental capabilities over a number of years – its impact is affected by what a person was like in the first place.

Personality, physical condition and social situation can all be important. Some people become increasingly disagreeable and difficult to live with, whereas others become more sweet-natured and amenable. Some people with Alzheimer's disease have few other health problems, whereas others have disabilities – such as arthritis or deafness – that can make their care more difficult. Some people have a comparatively comfortable social situation, whereas others are faced with family or financial problems.

How does Alzheimer's disease usually progress? Does it always follow the same course?

No two people with Alzheimer's disease will follow exactly the same course. The disease will progress more quickly in some people than in others; some people may die within five years, whilst others may live for more than 20 years after the diagnosis. Furthermore, no one will experience all of the symptoms and signs listed here. It is also important to note that the disease typically progresses gradually and does not fit neatly into the three stages outlined below. Even so, it can be helpful to look at the typical symptoms and signs of Alzheimer's disease in the context of three stages of development – early, middle and late. These stages will serve as a rough guide to the most likely progression of the disease and may help carers to be aware of potential problems and to make plans for future care needs.

Early symptoms
The early stage of Alzheimer's disease is often overlooked, being incorrectly labelled by professionals, relatives and friends as 'old age' or a normal part of the process of ageing. Because the onset of the disease is gradual, it is difficult to identify exactly when it begins. The person may:

- have difficulties with language;
- experience memory loss – having particular problems with short-term memory or memory for new things;
- be disorientated in time;
- become lost in familiar places;
- have difficulty in making decisions;
- lack initiative and motivation;
- show signs of depression and aggression;
- show a loss of interest in hobbies and activities.

Middle symptoms

As the disease progresses, problems become more evident and more restricting. The person with Alzheimer's disease has difficulty with day-to-day living, and is likely to:

- become very forgetful – especially of recent events and people's names;

- no longer manage to live alone without help;

- be unable to cook, clean or shop;

- need help with dressing;

- become extremely dependent;

- need assistance with personal hygiene, including using the toilet, bathing and washing;

- have some incontinence;

- have increased difficulty with speech;

- wander and sometimes gets lost;

- have various difficulties such as unprovoked aggression or constantly following their carer around the house;

- experience hallucinations (seeing or hearing things that are not there);

- become suspicious and paranoid;

- become depressed.

Late symptoms

This stage is one of increasing dependence and inactivity. Memory disturbances become more profound and the physical side of the disease becomes more obvious. The person is likely to:

- have difficulty eating;

- not recognise relatives, friends and familiar objects;
- have difficulty understanding and interpreting events;
- be unable to find his or her way around in the home;
- have difficulty walking;
- have bladder and bowel incontinence;
- be eventually confined to a wheelchair or bed.

Why is it that my wife, who has dementia, is able to remember things from years ago but can't remember what happened half an hour ago?

There are several linked processes involved in memory. First, an experience is perceived (i.e. recognised by the brain). It is then placed in a short-term memory store and retained for a brief time. If the experience recurs or is likely to be important, it goes into a long-term memory store. Finally, for a memory to be recaptured it must be recalled from the memory store.

People with dementia gradually lose the ability to enter new information into their memory store. They also have difficulty in recalling previously stored memories. Memory for recent events is affected first, which is why people with dementia tend to be better at recalling memories from long ago. Occasionally, when a recent memory has a lot of emotion attached to it (such as a bereavement), your wife may still remember this although she forgets many other recent things.

My wife no longer recognises me. Why is this?

This is a very painful experience that commonly occurs in the late stage of Alzheimer's disease. The likely explanation is that, although your wife may be able to see your face, she is unable to link this to her memories of you and therefore does not recognise you.

OUTLOOK

My doctor recently told me that my wife has Alzheimer's disease. Is it bound to get worse?

You will need to be prepared for a gradual worsening of your wife's condition over the years. Although there may be no apparent change between one month and the next, changes will be apparent between one year and the next. In general, most people with Alzheimer's disease become very forgetful and quite disabled within five to ten years or so of the diagnosis.

One way of helping your wife to live as well as possible as the disease progresses is to ensure that she receives prompt treatment for any other medical problems, such as depression (discussed in the section 'Treating symptoms' in Chapter 12) or an infection. Dementia drugs (see the section 'Drug treatments' in Chapter 12) may temporarily slow the progress of the symptoms for some people.

It is useful for relatives and carers to know about the likely progression of the disease so that they are aware of what is going to happen and can prepare themselves and make plans for the future. You will need to consider the possibility of day care, respite care (discussed in Chapter 9) and eventually residential care (see Chapter 10). Your doctor, community mental health nurse (formerly called community psychiatric nurse or CPN) or a member of a local carers' self-help group (such as a local Alzheimer's Society group) will be able to give you further advice.

3 | Getting a diagnosis

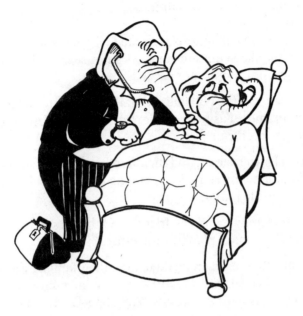

Alzheimer's disease and other dementias usually develop slowly and people may have been ill for some time before the diagnosis is thought of. Getting a diagnosis is important. If someone is diagnosed as having Alzheimer's disease or another dementia, they and their carers are better able to plan for the future and will be more prepared for what will happen.

Although there is no specific test for Alzheimer's disease, various tests and investigations can help indicate whether or not someone has the disease. This chapter explains some of the ways doctors try to diagnose dementia and decide whether the dementia is due to Alzheimer's disease or another cause. This chapter also explains some of the tests and investigations that may be used.

THE NEED FOR DIAGNOSIS

Why is diagnosis so important?

A proper medical diagnosis is needed whenever anyone develops dementia-like symptoms and does not seem to be getting any better. Diagnosis is important because:

- it can rule out the possibility that the symptoms have a different, more easily treatable, cause such as depression or a hormone problem;

- it provides the person and their family or friends with an explanation why someone is having memory problems or behaving differently;

- it allows family members, friends and the person with dementia to make plans for the future;

- it means that people with dementia, their families and carers can be provided with support and help, including some financial help (see the section 'State benefits' in Chapter 11);

- treatments are available that may help some of the symptoms; the sooner these treatments are started, the better.

I'm not sure, but I think my wife may be developing Alzheimer's disease. I have heard there is no cure, so is it necessary to involve the doctor?

You should definitely involve the doctor as soon as possible if you suspect that your wife may be developing Alzheimer's disease. There are several important reasons.

First, your wife may have a condition that looks like Alzheimer's disease but which is treatable. Examples include depression, under-activity of the thyroid gland or Parkinson's disease (these are discussed elsewhere in the book). Infections or constipation can also cause temporary confusion, as can some medicines such as strong painkillers, high blood pressure (hypertension) treatment or tranquillisers. Your wife's doctor will want to examine your wife and probably do some blood tests before coming to a diagnosis of dementia.

A second important reason to get a diagnosis is that this will help you and your wife to make plans for the future. For example, if it is found that your wife does have Alzheimer's disease, you should consider organising a Power of Attorney – called a Lasting Power of Attorney in the new Mental Capacity Act in England (discussed in Chapter 11) – while she is still able to do this. You will also be able to investigate the various types of help that may be available (see Chapter 9). It may also be necessary to discourage your wife from driving (see the section 'Driving' in Chapter 6).

Third, help and support including drug treatments may be available for your wife.

Is there any point in telling the difference between Alzheimer's disease and vascular dementia?

It can be difficult to determine whether a particular individual has Alzheimer's disease, vascular dementia (discussed in Chapter 1) or a mixture of the two. Furthermore, some doctors now believe that there is a lot of overlap between these two conditions. However, it is worth trying to tell the difference because this may affect how someone can best be looked after.

Alzheimer's disease and vascular dementia between them account for by far the greater majority of cases of dementia. If someone has a history of high blood pressure or stroke, or if a brain scan shows evidence of strokes in the brain, it is more likely that the person has vascular dementia. Another characteristic of this type of dementia is a more step-like progression, with the person suddenly developing new or worse symptoms from time to time, rather than the steadier decline that is typical of Alzheimer's disease.

If someone has vascular dementia, the doctor may want to prescribe aspirin or other drugs to thin the blood and try to prevent
further strokes. The doctor will also want to check the heart rhythm,
as sometimes an irregular heart beat can increase the risk of strokes.
If someone has Alzheimer's disease, especially if the disease is at an
early stage, they may be helped by one of the anti-dementia (anticholinesterase) drugs (see the section 'Drug treatments' in Chapter
12). Other treatments for memory impairment may also become
available in future.

My wife, who has Alzheimer's disease, seems to be very
withdrawn and increasingly forgetful. Is this due to the disease,
or might she also be suffering from depression? Can the doctor
do anything to help?

When someone has Alzheimer's disease or another dementia, it
can be very difficult to decide whether they are suffering from
depression as well. If you are worried that your wife may be
depressed, do tell her doctor.

Depression in someone with dementia may occur independently of
the dementia, or it may result from the dementia itself. Moodiness,
anxiety, fear and puzzlement are all understandable emotions in
people with dementia, especially early in the illness when they still
have some awareness of their failing capacities. Someone in your
wife's position will also be sensitive to the moods of the people
around her. If people with dementia become depressed, they often
cannot express these feelings in words. However, they may become
slow and withdrawn and appear more confused and forgetful. They
may also lose their appetite, causing loss of weight. Another thing
that can help tell whether your wife is depressed is to look at which
part of the day is best for her – people with dementia tend to be
brighter in the mornings, whereas people with depression may
improve as the day goes on.

It is certainly important to identify depression in someone with
dementia, because treating the depression (see 'Treating symptoms'

in Chapter 12) can help them feel better and make a significant contribution towards enabling them to make the best use of their failing mental abilities. Because so many symptoms of depression and dementia are the same, depression is hard to diagnose with certainty. Therefore, if your wife's doctor suspects depression as well as dementia, he or she may want to treat your wife with antidepressants to see whether she gets any better.

SEEKING A DIAGNOSIS

My husband has recently been showing disturbing signs of memory loss but won't see a doctor. Can you advise me?

Reluctance on the part of someone with memory problems to seek medical advice is common and understandable. Your husband may have no idea that anything is wrong, or alternatively he may fear that there is a problem but hopes that it will 'go away'.

If the difficulties have arisen quite suddenly – within weeks rather than months – seeking a medical opinion is a matter of urgency. If the loss of memory has been more gradual, the need for your husband to see a doctor is slightly less urgent. If at all possible, enlist his GP's help. He or she may well have developed a diplomatic way of overcoming this sort of problem. One possibility is for you to suggest to your husband that both of you ought to attend the doctor's surgery for a routine health check.

If for any reason the GP can't help, you could speak to your local Social Services or the Alzheimer's Society (contact details in Appendix 1) about the possibility of getting in touch directly with the psychiatric service that deals with problems of older people in your area.

Don't give up trying to persuade your husband to see a doctor – patience and perseverance generally pay. Your husband's mood and willingness to accept help may well vary from day to day. He may eventually agree on the grounds of saving you from worry.

When you do succeed in arranging for your husband to see a doctor, be prepared. Take time beforehand to draw up a written list of the problems, and of any questions you would like to be answered. If you are present when your husband is being interviewed, try not to interrupt or to prompt him. It is important for the doctor to be able to make his or her own independent assessment of your husband's condition. However, do ensure that you also have a time in which you can talk to the doctor without interruption.

I am sure my husband is starting with Alzheimer's disease. But every time I take him to our GP he puts on a show and convinces the doctor he is all right. Now the doctor has prescribed me tranquillisers! What can I do?

If you are really worried, you should seek further advice. It can sometimes be difficult to diagnose Alzheimer's disease in its early stages.

It is possible that you are right and your husband does have early Alzheimer's disease. However, many people become more forgetful as they get older without this amounting to Alzheimer's disease or progressing very much.

Before visiting the doctor again, it would probably be worth keeping a diary of your husband's symptoms. Nearly everyone forgets to say important things when they are sitting in front of the doctor, so writing them down first, either to read yourself or to show to the doctor, can be very helpful. If your GP has other partners in the practice, you could try speaking to one of them. You could also ask your husband's GP to refer your husband to a specialist for a second opinion. If your husband is able to 'put on a show' as you say, it may be worthwhile asking your GP to do a home visit, as seeing him at home can often give clues to the diagnosis.

Help! I have gone to my father's GP five times now, because my father is getting more and more confused. The GP says that confusion is a normal part of getting old, but I am sure Dad has Alzheimer's. I've tried talking to the practice manager but this has not helped. What can I do?

It is really important your father has a proper assessment. If you feel that your father is not getting the care he needs and the relationship with your father's GP has broken down, you may want to register your father with another practice. Details of GPs where your father lives can be found through your local Primary Care Trust, at local libraries or through the NHS website (see Appendix 1). Alternatively, if you contact your father's local Social Services for Older People, they may be able to help put you in touch with a specialist.

My father is 70 and clearly has a problem with his memory. He is Chairman of a Board of Directors and is quite unaware that he has a problem. I am very worried he will make a fool of himself. What can I do?

This is a very difficult situation. The possibilities are:

- His memory problems are just due to the usual decline in memory that people experience as part of getting older (see the section 'Symptoms and signs' in Chapter 2 for information on how dementia differs from normal forgetfulness).

- He is in the early stages of dementia.

- He is depressed.

- He has some other physical explanation for his apparent poor memory, such as deafness or Parkinson's disease.

The first step is to try to work out just how bad your father's memory is. Does he just have a problem remembering some names or appointments, or is the problem more widespread? In any event, you should probably try to persuade your father to see his doctor, and you should go along with him if you can.

If your father does not recognise that he has a problem, you may feel the need to talk to someone at his work. This will obviously be easier if you know any of his colleagues personally, but bear in mind that your father may be very upset or embarrassed if he thinks you are going behind his back.

Before taking this possibly drastic step, which could lead to his removal from the Board, you must ask yourself how much all this really matters. You may decide that it is reasonable to wait until one of his colleagues notices your father's difficulties and approaches either you or your father's doctor. On the other hand, if your father's work holds considerable responsibility and affects the lives of other people, you may need to take the initiative and talk to one of his colleagues sooner rather than later. This is something your father's GP could help with.

THE PROCESS OF DIAGNOSIS

How is Alzheimer's disease usually diagnosed?

A diagnosis of Alzheimer's disease is usually made on the basis of the person's symptoms and mental abilities. To obtain as much information as possible, the doctor will undertake a process known as 'history taking', during which he or she will talk to the patient, and probably also to someone else who knows the patient well, such as a family member or friend. There may also be a more formal assessment of a patient's physical and mental condition and needs (see the section 'Community care' in Chapter 9 for more information).

It is often difficult to make a conclusive diagnosis of Alzheimer's disease. Various other illnesses, such as depression, a thyroid problem, a vitamin deficiency or Parkinson's disease, can cause similar symptoms (these conditions are discussed elsewhere in this book). A full physical examination and various tests, including blood tests and perhaps a brain scan (see later in this chapter), can help rule out some of the other possibilities. If tests fail to show any other reason for a person's symptoms, the doctor will often make a diagnosis of Alzheimer's disease. Sometimes, the diagnosis is made only after observing how the patient's condition develops over a period of several months.

Is there a quick test for Alzheimer's disease? I think I read something about one in a magazine.

There is no simple, single, straightforward test for Alzheimer's disease. There have been some press reports about quick tests for Alzheimer's disease, but no reliable test exists at the present time.

Tests of various kinds, including blood tests and brain scans (see later in this chapter), can help doctors to rule out other possible causes of symptoms that resemble those of Alzheimer's disease, and in some cases a brain scan can give a clue that Alzheimer's is present. In the rare cases where Alzheimer's is passed on by a single gene, a genetic test (see later) will help confirm the diagnosis.

An absolutely certain diagnosis of Alzheimer's disease usually requires a post-mortem examination to look for the characteristic changes in brain tissue that occur in people with this disease (see the section 'Defining Alzheimer's disease' in Chapter 2 for more information). In practice, however, such examinations are rarely performed.

I am going to see the doctor because I think my mother may have Alzheimer's disease as she is so forgetful. What sort of things will the doctor want to know?

The doctor will want to know as much as possible about your mother's problem. You may find it useful to make some notes before the appointment. Try to remember when you first noticed your mother's forgetfulness. Also think about how it has progressed: did the problem occur suddenly or has it developed gradually over a period of time? Be ready to give some examples: for instance, does your mother:

- leave the cooker or taps on?

- forget to pay bills?

- lose the thread of conversations?

There may be many examples but you might not remember them all when you are with the doctor unless you write them down.

Unless the doctor already knows your mother quite well, he or she will want to ask you some details about your mother's life: for example, the type of work she does or did, the sort of person she is and what things she likes doing. The doctor might also want to ask you about aspects of your mother's medical history, including information about past illnesses and operations, and whether anyone else in the family has ever had Alzheimer's disease.

It would be very helpful for the doctor to see your mother. If she won't come with you to the surgery, you should ask her doctor whether he or she could visit your mother at home; a home visit from the doctor can be crucial in giving clues to the diagnosis. The doctor will want to examine your mother to assess her physical health and may also ask her some questions to test her memory.

The GP was unable to decide whether my wife has Alzheimer's disease and is making arrangements for her to see a specialist. What will this involve?

The exact procedure for involving a specialist in a possible case of Alzheimer's disease varies, depending on the GP and on which hospital consultant is approached. It is likely that your wife's GP will refer her to the local Older Adults Psychiatry Service. All consultants will want to ask about a patient's symptoms, in addition to the questions already asked by the GP.

Many consultants believe a first assessment is best done in the person's home. Your GP will advise you if this is to happen in your wife's case. A consultant who visits a patient at home will be able to pick up additional clues about the person's condition and will be able to assess how well or badly the person is coping in his or her home.

Other consultants prefer to see each patient, with a family member or friend, in a day hospital or clinic. You will be sent appointment details for your wife in due course if you have not already received them. The advantages of this approach are that it may be easier to conduct a thorough examination of the patient, that various investigations and tests can be carried out on the same day, and that a range of other professionals are on hand to help with the assessment.

If your wife is found to have Alzheimer's disease or one of the other dementias, a thorough assessment should extend beyond purely medical matters. It may cover, for example, how well she is able to cope in the home setting, your financial circumstances and whether Social Services are involved. A medical assessment is part of the 'needs assessment' that determines the types of community care that may be available (see the section 'Community care' in Chapter 9).

We went to the doctor because my husband is getting very forgetful. Now we have an appointment for a memory clinic. What is a memory clinic?

Memory clinics operate in different ways. The people who work there may include doctors, nurses, psychologists, occupational therapists and social workers, so it is difficult to generalise about the ways they work. However, if you attend a memory clinic you can expect that a doctor at the clinic will want to hear an account of the illness, both from your husband and from yourself. A psychologist may give your husband a special memory test (see below). An occupational therapist may assess your husband's abilities to manage around the home. Social workers will be able to advise you on how to deal with some of the implications of a diagnosis of dementia.

Sometimes, memory clinics are run by doctors who are conducting research into drugs that might prevent further memory problems. It is worth remembering that people with memory problems often need a wide range of assessment and that they need to be in touch with local Social Services. So if your husband has been referred to a memory clinic that is some distance away, it is important that you and he are not cut off from local services. You should discuss this with your husband's GP and with Social Services.

> *When the doctor told me that my wife has Alzheimer's disease I was so shocked that I didn't take in everything he said. What should I do?*

This is quite common. Don't be embarrassed about making an appointment to talk to the doctor again. It is important that you have a discussion about what your needs are, what sort of help is possible and what to expect in the future. It is also important that you try to ensure that there is some ongoing follow-up of both you and your wife, as the situation is inevitably going to change as time goes on. See whether you can be put in touch with a community nurse or Admiral nurse, who may be able to answer your questions. You could also call the Alzheimer's Society helpline for where you live – they can provide a lot of information for you (see Appendix 1 for contact details).

For the future, you might find it helpful to jot down information that the doctor or nurse gives you, so that you have it for future reference. There is a lot to take in.

MEMORY TESTS

> *My wife was visited by a psychiatrist and then a few weeks later by a community mental health nurse. Both did a test which I think was called the Mental State Examination. What is this and why do they do it, as it seems to distress my wife?*

The Mini Mental State Examination is one of a number of screening tests for dementia. It takes about five to six minutes to administer and involves asking people a set of questions to test their memory, orientation as to time and place, understanding and language ability. People taking the test are also asked to write a sentence and to copy a drawing.

The Mini Mental State Examination is commonly used by professionals caring for people with dementia. It is not a diagnostic test because the information it gives is not sufficient to allow a diagnosis of Alzheimer's disease or another dementia to be made. People can score low on the test for a number of different reasons. The test can, however, be useful for monitoring people's mental abilities in the early stages of dementia. Occasionally, people do get upset when they are asked apparently simple questions that they cannot answer or get wrong. If this happens, it may be better to leave things alone and return to the test later.

My partner has to see a psychologist next week for some kind of memory test. Can you explain why he needs to go and what will be involved?

Making a diagnosis of dementia can be quite difficult, especially when the illness is in its early stages. Furthermore, some people may complain of poor memory that is not obvious when the doctor first sees them. In these circumstances a doctor may decide to refer a patient to a clinical psychologist or to another doctor in order to have a more extensive set of memory tests.

Two commonly used tests are known as the Wechsler Adult Intelligence Scale and the Cambridge Cognitive Test (CAMCOG). Both of them take about an hour to complete. They are divided into a number of different sections and will test a variety of things, including the ability to learn new things and the ability to comprehend arithmetic and vocabulary. Such tests usually also include an assessment of physical skills, such as drawing and copying. These tests can be quite exhausting and the psychologist may suggest completing them over two appointments.

It is important to remember that these tests on their own cannot provide a diagnosis of dementia. Your partner's scores will be compared with what would be expected for a person of the same age and background, and even then can do no more than provide an indication of whether there is a problem.

BLOOD TESTS

The doctor recently did some blood tests on my wife, but didn't tell me what they were for. Is there a blood test for Alzheimer's disease?

Most cases of Alzheimer's disease cannot be diagnosed by a blood test. However, any person with symptoms that might be due to a dementia such as Alzheimer's disease is likely to be given various blood tests to make sure the symptoms don't have a treatable cause.

The blood tests normally include a check to ensure your wife is not anaemic or diabetic and a check of kidney and liver function, thyroid gland activity and calcium and vitamin levels in the blood. Occasionally, the doctor may check for the presence of syphilis or the HIV virus if this is thought necessary. The genetic test (see below) for the rare inherited cases of Alzheimer's disease (see the section 'Who will get Alzheimer's disease?' in Chapter 2) takes the form of a blood test.

Do not be afraid to ask the doctor about any tests that he or she might do with your wife.

My partner, a man of 40, is becoming very forgetful. His doctor wants him to have an HIV test. I am sure that my partner has been faithful and that he does not have HIV. Is the test really necessary?

Any type of dementia at the age of 40 is extremely uncommon and requires thorough investigation. Infection with HIV (human immunodeficiency virus) is one possible cause of dementia in younger people. This virus, which is associated with AIDS (acquired immune deficiency syndrome), can enter the brain and cause problems of its own accord, or it can result in other disorders affecting the brain, such as fungal infections. Some people with HIV infection or AIDS do develop a form of dementia (see the section 'Types of dementia' in Chapter 1 for more information).

Some doctors recommend an HIV test only if they think that a patient is at particular risk of HIV infection – for example, a gay man, someone who shares needles when injecting drugs, or someone who has received blood or blood products abroad. Other doctors recommend an HIV test simply because they want to make sure they have considered every possible type of dementia, especially in a younger person such as your partner. All people who are considering having an HIV test should first receive counselling.

If an HIV test is performed and turns out to be positive, it means that appropriate treatment can be given without delay. Drugs can be prescribed to slow down the progress of AIDS. Also, knowing that someone is HIV-positive enables doctors to keep a look out for other conditions commonly associated with AIDS, such as fungal infections, and to treat these early.

It is also useful for doctors to know that a younger patient with dementia is HIV-negative. Having ruled out HIV as a possible cause of the dementia, they can move on to more extensive investigations to try to find out the actual cause.

GENETIC TESTS

My grandmother, father and uncle all developed Alzheimer's disease around the age of 50. It seems that our family may have a rare inherited form of the disease. I've been offered a genetic test, but don't know whether to have it. What are the advantages and disadvantages?

This is a complex question and it is better to talk the issues through with a trained counsellor and a doctor who specialises in genetic diseases. Don't be hurried into a decision.

If you do have the test, which is a simple blood test, it will show whether or not you are carrying the gene that has caused Alzheimer's disease in your family. If your father had the gene, you have a one in two chance of having inherited it. If you do have the gene, you will almost certainly develop Alzheimer's disease at around the same age as the other members of your family. If you don't have the gene, this is very unlikely.

The disadvantages of the test are that, if it shows that you do have the gene, you may have difficulty getting life insurance, a mortgage or even a job if you declare that you have had it. If you know that you have the gene but fail to declare this information, any insurance you take out is likely to be invalid. You may also find it hard to cope with the knowledge that you will develop a disease for which there is no cure. On the other hand, you may prefer to know what to expect, so that you can plan your life accordingly. You may also be wondering about having children and want to know if you are at risk of passing on the gene to them. Before you make any decisions, talk this through with a genetic counsellor, whom you can contact through your GP.

My father had Alzheimer's disease, diagnosed when he was 70.
I know there is a gene test for Alzheimer's. Should I have it?

The answer is almost certainly no. If family members have the very rare form of Alzheimer's disease carried by a single gene (see 'Who will get Alzheimer's disease?' in Chapter 2), it usually develops when they are in their 40s or 50s.

Although genes may play some part in the development of Alzheimer's disease in people who develop it later in life, genes are not thought to cause the disease as they do the early-onset type of the illness. Genes probably play only a small part in the development of this much more common later-onset Alzheimer's disease.

Because your father has the later-onset form of the disease, the role of genes in his illness is less clear-cut and no tests exist yet for these genes. With further research, more 'dementia genes' may be identified in the future.

Even in cases where genetic tests are available, there are good reasons for being cautious. Before having any such tests, you need to consider whether the result will be helpful to you. A positive test may stop you from getting life insurance, a mortgage or even a job. It may affect your relationship. You may also have years of worry about developing something that you cannot prevent.

In future, if better treatments for Alzheimer's disease become available, there may be more point in having genetic tests if these become available.

BRAIN SCANS

My doctor has diagnosed my mother as having Alzheimer's
disease, but has not done a brain scan. Isn't a brain scan
necessary in every case?

In fact the usual type of brain scan (a CT scan, see below) is of limited use in diagnosing Alzheimer's disease and most other dementias. All the brain scan is likely to show is some shrinkage of the brain, but this can occur in people who do not have dementia. Also, an entirely normal scan does not rule out the possibility of dementia.

The main reasons for doing a brain scan are if a patient's symptoms are not typical or if the doctor suspects a brain tumour. A brain tumour is rarely a cause of dementia, and other symptoms and findings when the doctor examines the patient would be likely to suggest this diagnosis. Brain scans can also point to whether someone has vascular dementia (see the section 'Types of dementia' in Chapter 1) rather than Alzheimer's disease, but again this information is often apparent from a person's medical history. Most doctors now prefer to do MRI scans (discussed later in this section), which can provide better images of the brain although these take a lot longer and are not available everywhere.

What is the difference between a CT scan and a CAT scan?

There is no difference. The terms CT scan and CAT scan are both abbreviations for Computed Axial Tomography. (See the next answer for details.)

My wife is having a CT scan of her brain. What does this involve?

A CT scan is a way of taking pictures of the brain using X-rays and a computer. The result is a series of computer-generated pictures that show 'slices' of the brain. CT scans are useful for diagnosing strokes and tumours. They may also show changes, such as thinning of the brain tissue, that occur in people with Alzheimer's disease. CT scans can also help doctors to distinguish between vascular dementia and Alzheimer's disease.

A CT scan will normally be performed on an out-patient basis, with the scan itself taking only a few minutes. Some people find the procedure rather disturbing and may not be able to stay still long enough. If a scan is considered to be absolutely necessary for someone who is likely to become agitated, he or she may be given a light sedative. An injection into the bloodstream may be given to help show the brain more clearly.

The CT scanner looks a bit like a very large front-loading washing machine. It may be in a room with a lot of equipment and may look a little daunting at first. Your wife will be asked to lie on a narrow bed with her head near the scanner entrance. The scan will be performed by a radiographer, who will operate the controls from an adjacent room and will watch your wife through a large window. The bed on which your wife is lying will move into the scanner, and a series of X-rays will be taken. There is a little noise.

At the end, there will be a series of about 20 pictures showing your wife's brain from top to bottom. If your wife is given a sedative, you will have to wait for the effects to wear off. Otherwise, you will be able to go home immediately after the scan. The radiographer will not be able to give you any results. These will take a few days because the films from the scan need to be examined closely.

What is an MRI scan? Is it better than a CT scan?

MRI stands for Magnetic Resonance Imaging. Like CT scans, MRI scans use a computer to create pictures of 'slices' through the brain. But unlike CT scans, MRI scans do not use X-rays to obtain the image. Instead, they use radio signals produced by the body in response to the effects of a very strong magnet contained within the scanner. Because of this magnet, it is important not to wear anything metal, including jewellery, when having an MRI scan. It is also important to tell the doctor or technician if you have anything metal inside your body (such as a pacemaker). MRI scans show more detail than CT scans but they take longer to do and are more expensive. Sometimes a doctor will ask for an MRI scan if the CT scan doesn't show enough information.

Like CT scanners, MRI scanners look like large washing machines: the hole in the middle is the scanner entrance. MRI scans are quite noisy, and can take up to an hour to do. It is essential that the person having the scan remains very still throughout; this can cause some discomfort, so it is important to be really comfortable before the scanning begins.

I took my partner to see a specialist and he ordered a SPECT scan. What is this?

SPECT stands for Single Photon Emission Computed Tomography. This type of scan, unlike a CT scan or an MRI scan, looks at blood flow through the brain, rather than at the structure of the brain. Research suggests that the information provided by a SPECT scan may help in confirming the diagnosis of dementia in some cases. Also, different types of SPECT scans can help tell whether someone has Alzheimer's disease, vascular dementia or Lewy body dementia.

A SPECT scan is very simple. The person to be scanned is first given an injection of a very mild radioactive substance, which is quite safe. This substance (a radionuclide) travels in the blood to the brain. The person then has to sit still while the scanner, which looks like a rotating hair dryer, takes pictures of the brain. The result is a series of computer-generated pictures of 'slices' of the brain. These slices are like a map. They show variations in the amount of radionuclide that is taken up by the brain. This in turn shows how well the blood is flowing to different areas in the brain.

TALKING ABOUT THE DIAGNOSIS

My wife has just been diagnosed with Alzheimer's disease. Should she be told the diagnosis, and who should tell her?

Although you may think it will be painful and difficult for your wife, it may be for the best if she is told the diagnosis. Most doctors now tell most people with dementia their diagnosis, and probably the first step should be for you to talk this through with your wife's doctor or specialist. There are a number of advantages if your wife is informed about the diagnosis:

- She may be able to understand why she is having problems with her memory.

- She may be able to plan for the future with you; for example, by making legal and financial arrangements (discussed in Chapter 11) or taking a holiday.

- It may be possible to discuss and plan treatment with a dementia drug (see the section 'Drug treatments' in Chapter 12).

- There will be no need for secrecy in the family.

To a certain extent, whether your wife is told the diagnosis depends on how advanced the Alzheimer's disease is. If your wife is told her diagnosis, it is important that she (and you) are given proper support and counselling after this. Many GPs have practice counsellors, or your local Old Age Psychiatry Service may be able to help here. (See also Chapter 9 for information on getting help and support.) It is worth remembering that your wife may find being given the diagnosis very painful or upsetting. Also, she may not believe it initially (denial is a natural reaction) or she may not remember it later. In both these circumstances, a gentle persuasive approach is better than confrontation.

My husband, who has Alzheimer's disease, gets upset when he forgets things. Should I remind him about his diagnosis, so that he can understand what is happening to him?

Some people in the early stages of Alzheimer's disease seem to appreciate that their memory is failing. Gently reminding them of the reason for this may help them feel less pressured and so reduce stress. However, as time goes on, people who have Alzheimer's disease become generally unaware of their problems. Reminding someone with more advanced Alzheimer's disease that their memory is failing is unlikely to help them to understand their condition and may add to their distress.

My mother, who lives with us, has been diagnosed with Alzheimer's disease. I have been so worried about her that I have not been able to work out what to tell my children. They realise there is something wrong with their grandmother. What should I say?

Children are very resilient and generally respond well to being told the truth. Explain the facts to them as clearly as you can, and give them plenty of opportunity to ask questions. You should have this conversation with them as soon as possible because they may be blaming themselves for their grandmother's strange behaviour. Finding out that it is due to an illness is likely to be a relief to them. This is a difficult time for all of you. The best way of helping your children to cope with it is to give them plenty of explanations, reassurance, hugs and love. There are also a few books that have been written for children and young people on the subject of Alzheimer's disease (see Appendix 2), and the Alzheimer's Society (contact details in Appendix 1) has a leaflet for teenagers.

4 | Practical care day to day

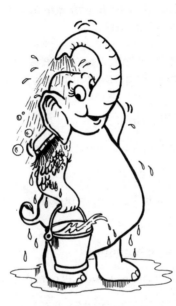

Activities such as dressing, washing, using the toilet, eating and sleeping are a normal part of everyday life. However, even these routine tasks become increasingly difficult for people with dementia to perform on their own. This chapter provides some useful guidelines as to how people with dementia and carers might be able to help the people themselves to live as well and as independently as possible. The amount of help needed will obviously change over time.

GENERAL QUESTIONS

My father, who has Alzheimer's disease, is coming to live with me and my family. I fear he is going to be difficult to look after, so can you give me any tips?

It can be difficult to look after someone with Alzheimer's disease. However, you may find the following tips from other carers helpful:

- Try to establish a routine.
- Allow your father some independence.
- Help him maintain his dignity.
- Avoid confrontation whenever possible.
- Keep tasks simple.
- Maintain a sense of humour.
- Make sure your home is as safe as possible.
- Encourage your father to take exercise.
- Help make the best of your father's existing abilities.
- Remember that problems are probably due to the disease, not the person.
- At all times be flexible, because dementia is progressive, and you are both going to have to adapt with the changes that occur as time goes on.
- Learn as much as possible about his condition.
- Keep in touch with other carers.
- Recognise when the strain on you and your family is becoming too much.

My husband has recently been diagnosed as having Alzheimer's disease. I am in my early 70s and still very fit. How long am I likely to be able to carry on looking after him in our home?

The answer to this question will depend on the rate at which your husband's illness progresses, on your own on-going state of health and on how much support you can get from family, friends and outside agencies. (See Chapter 9 for information on getting help.) Even with support, though, you are unlikely to be able to manage your husband at home in the later stages of his illness. However, it is not really possible to predict in advance how long it will be before this point is reached.

Do you think it is possible that my wife with dementia is able to do less and less for herself because I am doing more and more for her?

Your wife is able to do less and less because dementia is a progressive condition. This means that her abilities will inevitably decline with time. You will need to do more and more for her as time goes on, but if you do too much for her too soon her abilities will decline more rapidly.

It is important to recognise the things that your wife can still do for herself and to encourage her to do these even though she may take a long time to do them. If you disregard what she is still capable of, and do everything for her, she will quickly lose the functions that she still has. Try to be patient and to take over from her only the things that she really can no longer manage. The progressive nature of the disease means that the situation will continue to change. You will be able to respond best to your wife's changing needs if you work with her, and are flexible in your attitudes.

My mother has Alzheimer's disease. She also has painful-looking
leg ulcers. She doesn't complain about them. Can people with
dementia feel pain?

It can be quite difficult to know how much pain someone with
Alzheimer's disease or another dementia is experiencing. This is
particularly true later in the illness, when not only are people unable
to tell you that they are in pain but also even their normal responses
to pain can be difficult to interpret.

Recognising that someone is in pain is less of a problem earlier in
the illness, particularly if you are looking after someone you have
known for a long time. You will usually be able to tell that something is wrong from the way that the person behaves. For example,
he or she may become restless, sleep badly or not want to eat. Also
look out for changes in their posture or gait or changes in their facial
expressions. However, even though you may recognise that the person is in pain, you will not be able to rely on him or her to tell you
where the pain is or how severe it may be. You (or the doctor) will
have to work this out from what you know about the person.

In general, it is best to assume that a procedure that would normally be painful – such as having a leg ulcer dressed – would be
equally painful for someone who has dementia, even though they
cannot tell you about it.

DRESSING

We both want my husband to carry on dressing himself for as
long as possible. However, he is finding it increasingly difficult.
Can you suggest how I might be able to make dressing easier
for him?

You are right to continue to encourage your husband to dress.
One way of helping your husband is to make sure that he
always has plenty of time. Provided that the room is warm, it does

not matter if dressing takes a while. It might also help him to manage better if you lay his clothes out for him in the order he needs to put them on. Later in the illness, you will probably need to hand his clothes to him one at a time, and give instructions as to how to put them on.

Some clothes are easier to put on than others. Neck openings should be a good size. Raglan or drop sleeves are easier than tight sleeves. Slip-on shoes are useful. Clothes with elasticated openings or Velcro fastenings are simpler than clothes fastened with buttons. Some people find that T-shirts and track suits are an excellent substitute for ordinary shirts, trousers and jackets. However, if your husband has been used to wearing more traditional clothing in the past, he may not like the change. If at all possible, do try to involve him in choosing what he is going to wear each day.

I have early dementia. I'm having real difficulty deciding what to wear and seem to end up with the same clothes each day. The wardrobe is too full of choice for me.

It is very common to have too many clothes in your wardrobe, which you have had for years but cannot bear to part with. Try to go through what you have and pick the clothes you really like. Be brave, throw or give away the rest. You might need some help with this, so ask a relative or close friend to do it with you.

I'm having real problems persuading my mother not to wear the same clothes for days on end. Her clothes get really grubby and she often looks unkempt. She gets so upset if I say anything. What can I do?

Your mother probably no longer recognises the need to change her clothes nor knows which ones are clean and which need washing. One possible way to help might be to encourage her to have a bath and then take this opportunity to remove the clothes that need washing and to lay out a clean set for her. If you do this, she will probably put the clothes on and you will not be hurting her feelings.

PERSONAL HYGIENE

Is it common for people with Alzheimer's disease to hate having their faces washed? My wife does not mind having a bath, but protests at having her face washed. Does it matter?

This is not especially common. What has probably happened is that your wife no longer understands the need to wash her face. She may also find it undignified to have someone else wash her face for her. Of course, it does not really matter if her face is not washed. It certainly is not worth having a battle about this.

You could try buying a new soft and pretty flannel. Then try to make face washing fun by getting your wife to wash your face with it before she either lets you wash her face or does it herself.

My husband is always washing his hands. He seems to forget he's just done it. The main problem is that he keeps leaving the taps running. How can I stop him from flooding the bathroom?

Various tap adaptations are available. Some will cause water to flow only when someone's hands are under them. Others have an automatic cut-off after a certain quantity of water has been run, or after a set time. Your water company should be able to provide a catalogue. These adaptations may seem expensive, but if you have metered water will probably save you money as well as much mopping up. If you can't afford the adaptation, it may be worth trying your local Social Services or the caring fund of your local Alzheimer's Society branch.

An alternative approach, if you haven't already tried it, is to find other activities for your husband that may distract him from the repetitive washing activity.

How can I make it safer to give my mother a bath?

Bath time can be dangerous, especially for elderly, frail people with dementia. Bathrooms are slippery places, and it can be very difficult to lift someone when they are wet. Use non-slip mats in the bath and on the bathroom floor. Always put cold water into the bath before adding hot, and remember that the skin of an older person is much more sensitive to temperature. You may also need special rails or a bath seat (a device that rests in the bath for a person to sit on). Speak to your mother's doctor or Social Services about obtaining these aids. An occupational therapist can then visit your home to assess your mother's particular needs. It may also be possible to arrange for a care assistant or nurse (see see the section on the section on Community care in Chapter 9) to come and give your mother a bath.

My husband, who has Alzheimer's, is very reluctant to take a bath or shower and his personal hygiene is suffering as a result. Can you advise me please?

Personal hygiene frequently requires tact and diplomacy. If reminders of the need to take a bath or shower are no longer effective, establishing a regular routine will help him to carry out the tasks involved. When his motivation slips, try to ensure that he has a regular event for which it is worth being well groomed – for example, going to the day centre or visiting a friend or the pub.

Lots of praise and encouragement when he is freshly bathed and dressed is far more valuable than constant criticism about his cleanliness. If your husband is not able to carry out the task of bathing alone, try not to take over more than is absolutely necessary. He may be able to do everything needed to have a bath but might need help to do it in the right order.

It is possible that your husband may respond favourably to being given a degree of choice over bathing. For example, you could ask him whether he wants a bath first thing in the morning or last thing at night. Alternatively, he might accept being told that a warm bath has been run for him as he 'usually has one before bed'. Some carers have found that asking the person if they want a hot drink 'before or after their bath' can be effective. Ensure that the bathroom is warm, and minimise any impression that bathing is a chore.

Some older people never or rarely bath or shower, preferring a good strip-down wash. If this has been your husband's preference in the past, it is better to build on this rather than try to impose a new system.

When I am helping my elderly father, who has Alzheimer's disease, to undress or take a bath, he often shouts 'rape' and tries to push me away.

For many people, undressing and bathing have always been private functions, and it is quite possible that this is what your father believes. He may also find it very odd that he now has to have help with these things. It is also possible that he no longer recognises you and may see you as a stranger invading his privacy.

If your father becomes agitated when you try to bath him, the best thing to do is to abandon the attempt for another time. If the problem continues, it might be worth asking for a nurse to come in and bath him. Alternatively, it might be possible, if your father goes to a day centre, to arrange for him to be given a bath or shower while he is there.

Is it common for people with Alzheimer's disease to become incontinent? Is their incontinence caused mainly by confusion, or are there other reasons?

Many people with Alzheimer's disease are occasionally incontinent, especially of urine. Often, confusion is the main cause, but there are other possibilities to be aware of. It is sensible to consult the doctor if someone becomes incontinent, because treatment of the cause may be possible.

If incontinence of urine comes on suddenly, or if the urine has an unpleasant smell or is dark in colour, the problem may be a bladder infection. It should be possible for a doctor to treat such an infection with drugs.

Other treatable causes of incontinence of urine include enlargement of the prostate gland in men, and severe constipation, both of which can interfere with the normal flow of urine. Severe constipation can also cause incontinence of faeces, when semi-solid faecal matter leaks around an impacted faecal mass, making it look as though the person has diarrhoea when in fact the opposite is the problem.

The use of certain medicines can also contribute to incontinence. Sedatives and tranquillisers, for example, often reduce the sensation of needing to pass urine and also slow down the instinct to get to the toilet. Diuretics (water pills), which may be needed to treat another problem, may make incontinence more likely by increasing urine production.

My husband, diagnosed with Alzheimer's disease, has begun to wet the bed. What can I do?

If you have not already done so, speak to your husband's GP as the incontinence may be treatable, at least to some extent (see the previous answer). If your husband's bed-wetting is due mainly to increased confusion, there are a number of practical steps that you can take to reduce the problem.

Try to ensure that he does not have large drinks last thing at night. Also cut down on tea and coffee, which increase urine output by their diuretic action. Encourage your husband to go to the toilet before he goes to bed. You may find it helpful to wake him once or twice during the night for a toilet visit. Also consider whether the toilet is near enough to the bedroom. Older people may have no time to waste looking for the toilet. Make sure he is confident in finding the toilet and managing the door. Some carers find that little night-lights that plug into wall sockets help; if they are in the right place, they can help to guide the person to the loo, and help to prevent trips and falls.

You could also consider the use of a commode or bed bottle. A waterproof mattress cover would be useful. The district nurse should be able to advise you and to lend you appropriate equipment. He or she should also know about other possible sources of local help, such as Incontact, which provides advice on continence problems (see Appendix 1).

I'm at the end of my tether. My wife has Alzheimer's disease. She keeps wetting herself. Now I'm afraid to take her out. What can I do?

First check with your wife's doctor that her incontinence does not have a treatable cause (discussed earlier in this section), such as a bladder infection. If no treatable cause for the incontinence is found, the following practical steps may help.

Try to remind your wife to go to the toilet when she gets up in the morning, every couple of hours during the day and last thing at night. If she empties her bladder often, there may be fewer accidents. You may also notice signs that mean she needs to go to the toilet: for example, she may fidget or pace around. If this happens, prompt her to go to the toilet. Ensure that the toilet is easily accessible, warm and well lit.

Incontinence pads will soak up small volumes of urine and can give you both confidence to leave the house. These come in different varieties and it's worth speaking to a continence adviser about them. Other things to consider include having waterproof covers for your wife's usual chair, car seat and mattress. Continence advisers will have various ideas that may help you. Your GP should be able to put you in touch.

Incontinence can lead to sore skin, so your wife will need bathing or showering at least daily. In between times, it may be necessary to clean her with baby wipes. If your wife's skin does become red and sore, speak to her doctor: your wife may have a fungal infection that can be easily treated with the right cream.

Incontinence will mean a lot more work for you. Many people find it upsetting and distasteful. You may begin to feel angry and bitter.

This is very understandable, but do try to talk to people about the problem and about your feelings. Your GP, hospital specialist, district nurse, social worker and continence adviser will all have come across this before and will be able to help.

My mother has developed a habit of putting pieces of used toilet paper down the back of the bathroom radiator. When I ask her about this, she denies that she has done it. How should I handle this?

It seems that your mother has forgotten what to do with the toilet paper she has used. She may also have forgotten how to flush the toilet. It is unlikely to be useful to confront her with what she is doing. If possible, stand outside the bathroom door and when you think she is ready, go in and help her to flush her used paper down the toilet.

When we are out driving, getting my wife to the toilet can be quite a problem, especially as I can't just take her to the door and leave her. What is the best thing to do if she needs to use a public toilet?

Many carers face this problem. The best thing to do is to use the disabled people's toilets, which are now available in most public buildings. You will find that these toilets are large enough for you to go in with your wife and assist her if that is necessary.

In some places, such as motorway service stations and multi-storey car parks, the disabled toilets are often kept locked. These are often accessed with a key that you can obtain from RADAR (contact details in Appendix 1). Otherwise, the key will usually be available either from the kiosk or the information desk. RADAR also produces a guide to the location of RADAR toilets around the UK. Armed with this, you can plan your journeys safe in the knowledge that there is a toilet you can use en route.

Sometimes, the disabled toilet is inside the Ladies or Gents. If it is inside the Ladies, the only option is to be bold enough to go in there with your wife. You will find that most people will be understanding and discreet. If you are challenged, you have a good answer of course.

FOOD AND DRINK

My wife has only a very small appetite and often refuses to eat anything at all. How can I persuade her? Is it usual for someone with Alzheimer's disease not to want to eat?

This is a common problem in the later stages of Alzheimer's disease. It is quite possible that your wife no longer understands about eating what is put in front of her. She may not feel hungry, perhaps because she takes very little exercise, or she may no longer recognise what it is to be hungry. It is also possible that your wife is having problems chewing or swallowing (see later in this section).

Try to make mealtimes part of a calm, relaxed routine. Encourage your wife to eat, and praise her when she succeeds. Suggest that she might find it easier to use a spoon instead of a knife and fork. Or give her finger food if she prefers this. Do not criticise her if she makes a mess (see the answer later in this section). If she has problems chewing and swallowing, it may be simplest to liquidise her food. If she is very forgetful, you may need to prompt her to take another mouthful, or to chew or swallow it.

However, the most important thing is that, even if your wife does not want to eat, you should try to make sure that she drinks enough liquids – approximately eight cups a day is a rough guide. Plenty of liquid prevents constipation and dehydration, both of which can make confusion worse.

The Alzheimer's Society has a book *Food for Thought*, which includes other helpful tips for dealing with this problem (see Appendix 2).

My mother, who has had Alzheimer's disease for some years now, still has a good appetite but has lost a great deal of weight and is now very thin. Is this loss of weight due to her Alzheimer's disease? Do you think I should give her vitamin supplements?

It does seem that loss of weight may be a feature of Alzheimer's disease, although more research is needed into this.

It is sometimes helpful to give vitamin supplements to people in the later stages of dementia, but it would be best to speak to your mother's doctor first. He or she will be able to advise you on which supplements, if any, might be best for your mother.

My husband, who has Alzheimer's disease, sometimes forgets that he has just had a meal. He then complains about being hungry and says I never give him anything to eat. What can I do?

It is quite common for people who are confused to forget they have just had a meal. An added problem may be that your husband no longer knows when he has had enough to eat – probably because the disease has affected the part of the brain that tells him he is full.

If your husband asks for another meal when he has just eaten, the best plan is to try to distract him with some other activity. If this fails, you could offer him a snack, such as a piece of fruit, raw carrot or a stick of celery, to eat 'while he is waiting'. With luck, he will then forget that he was wanting a meal.

Why does my wife, who has Alzheimer's disease, want to eat sweets and chocolates all the time?

It may be that your wife's disease has affected a particular part of the brain that normally helps people control their intake of sweet things. Alternatively, it may just be that your wife has always been extremely fond of sweets and chocolates, but used to be able to resist them. Try offering her fresh or dried fruits instead.

*I am caring for my elderly father, who has recently been
diagnosed with Alzheimer's disease. He seems to be very prone
to constipation. Can you advise?*

You should try to ensure that your father eats a balanced diet
containing plenty of dietary fibre. He will do this more readily if
you offer him foods that he likes. Foods that have a high fibre
content include wholemeal bread and pasta, bran, cereals, pulses
and dried fruits.

One simple way of increasing the fibre content in the diet is to add
bran to cereals, stewed fruit and puddings. Your father should also
be encouraged to eat plenty of fresh fruit and vegetables, which will
provide him with vitamins as well as fibre. Drinking plenty of liquid
during the day will also help guard against constipation, as will taking plenty of exercise.

If your father is unwilling to eat the foods that would be good for
him, and continues to suffer from constipation, his doctor will probably be able to help. It is important to treat constipation in someone
with Alzheimer's disease because constipation can cause agitation
and aggravate confusion. The doctor may advise taking a laxative
such as ispaghula (e.g. Regulan or Fybogel), which contains added
fibre, or lactulose, which is a different sort of laxative that can also be
very effective. Any of these laxatives (but not some of the others that
are available over the counter) can be taken daily without harmful
effect. In a small number of cases, it may be necessary for a district
nurse to come and give regular enemas.

*If my wife, who has Alzheimer's disease, wants to eat baked
beans out of the tin; is there anything wrong in it?*

No, there is nothing wrong. Caring for someone with Alzheimer's
disease requires people to be flexible about eating habits. Do
make sure, however, that the tin has only just been opened, so that
the beans are fresh. Also make sure, if your wife is feeding herself,
that she does not cut herself on the opened tin.

My mother can no longer use a knife and fork properly and makes a dreadful mess. I find this very difficult to manage. Can you advise?

It is important for your mother's sense of independence and self-esteem that you encourage her to continue to feed herself for as long as possible. However, both you and she will probably find this frustrating at times.

Try always to be as flexible and tolerant as possible, and remember that your mother cannot help her table manners. She will probably cope best if you can make mealtimes as relaxed and unhurried as possible. It will also help her if you praise her for eating and enjoying her food, rather than getting upset about the mess.

Cleaning up afterwards will be easier if you use a plastic table cloth. If your mother can't cope with a table napkin, you could encourage her to wear an easily washable apron or smock when she eats. Try tactfully to encourage her to use a spoon rather than a knife and fork, but do make sure that the food is cut up well for her. Finger food is a good alternative. She will find it much easier to pick up food with her fingers. Examples of finger foods include chicken nuggets, scotch eggs, small pieces of cheese, muffins or toast with whatever she likes on it.

To reduce confusion, it is a good idea to serve only one portion of food at a time. Also, if possible, remove salt, pepper and sauces from the table as soon as they have been used.

It may be worth asking if an occupational therapist can call to give you further advice. Aids that might possibly be helpful include non-slip mats, plates with suction pads, plate guards and cutlery with easy-grip handles.

Why has my partner, who has dementia, suddenly become a vegetarian? He used to love meat.

A possible reason is that he no longer recognises meat for what it is, and that he finds it difficult to chew and swallow compared with some softer foods. (See also the next answer.) Being a vegetarian will do him no harm.

> *I have dementia and I seem to take ages to eat now. Meat and chewy food gets cold before I can finish it. I much prefer softer food now. What options are there for my husband and me, apart from mince?*

Food that you can break up easily with the side of a fork will be easy to chew. Some examples are scrambled eggs, fish or fishcakes in a sauce, well cooked pasta in a smooth sauce. Mashed potatoes, parsnip, mushy peas, bananas or stewed fruit are all easy to eat.

> *My wife, who has had Alzheimer's for some time now, finds chewing and swallowing a great problem. I find it very upsetting and I just don't know what to do.*

Problems with chewing and swallowing do sometimes occur in the later stages of Alzheimer's disease and can be very upsetting. The most likely cause is that the muscles and reflexes involved in chewing and swallowing are no longer working so well. Sometimes, however, a person's chewing problems are due simply to ill-fitting dentures or sore gums, which can be sorted out. It might be useful to ask for professional advice.

The most important thing for you to try to accept is that your wife needs only a very small amount of food. Soft and mashable foods at regular intervals, together with plenty to drink, will probably be quite adequate.

If you can manage to be reasonably relaxed about all this, and can help your wife to take sufficient food for her needs, you do not risk subjecting her to more undignified, uncomfortable and even hazardous methods of feeding.

*My husband, who has dementia, was formerly a strict
one-drink-before-supper man. Now he makes too many visits
to the drinks cupboard, with disastrous results. If I remove the
bottles, he is still capable of going out to buy more. What should
I do?*

It seems that your husband has always liked to drink in moderation and it will probably be best for him if he is able to continue this habit.

The most likely reason for your husband's present drinking problem is that he forgets when he has already had a drink and so has another. You may need to be fairly imaginative in dealing with this, for example by having only a few bottles, each with only a little in them, and topping them up yourself when they are empty. Perhaps you could ask people working in the local shop not to sell him alcohol.

At the same time, it is reasonable to offer him a drink with his main meal each day. It might also be worth bearing in mind that he could be bored and might drink less if you can find him some distracting activities (see Chapter 5 for information about activities).

KEEPING HEALTHY

*What can I and my carer do to keep ourselves physically fit
and well?*

It is important to have a good balanced diet, drink plenty of liquids, to take regular exercise, not to smoke, and to drink alcohol in moderation only. Walking is the best exercise: try to go out morning and afternoon. If you can't go out, even doing stretching or flexibility exercises in your chair will be helpful.

Check with your GP that any tablets you are on really are necessary. Medicines sometimes have side effects that can make you feel worse rather than better. Have regular checks of your eyes, hearing and oral health.

I feel low all the time and quite frightened. What can I do?

Y ou are probably feeling depressed. Depression is treatable. You might want to consider talking to your GP about how you are feeling. Your GP may then refer you to a qualified counsellor. Support from family and friends can also help you. Try to maintain your interests and be useful to other people – this will help to build up your confidence. If these things don't work, you may want to consider discussing with your GP taking anti-depressant pills.

TAKING PILLS

I have been prescribed tablets for my Alzheimer's disease, but I'm worried I'll forget to take them. What can I do?

Y ou have probably been prescribed one of the drugs developed to treat Alzheimer's disease (see 'Drug treatments' in Chapter 12). These drugs need to be taken at least daily in order to have a chance of improving your condition.

If someone can prompt you to take your tablets every day, even by a telephone call, this could help. Another possibility is to use a compartmentalised box, such as a Dosette or Medidose box. These boxes, which are available from chemist/pharmacist shops, have a different compartment for each day of the week. You, or your carer if you have one, could then help yourself by popping the tablets into a compartment for each day at the beginning of the week. Use of such a box might prompt you to take your medication. It will also provide you with an easy way of knowing whether or not you have already taken a tablet.

My husband is on a number of different tablets from the doctor. I am not sure what they are all for, but I have great difficulty getting him to swallow them all, especially the very large ones. What should I do?

It is quite common for people with dementia to be reluctant to take tablets. The problem usually occurs because people fail to recognise that there is anything wrong with them, and so do not appreciate the need to take medication. A problem with swallowing pills also sometimes occurs in the later stages of dementia as part of a more general difficulty with swallowing (see the section 'Drug treatments' in Chapter 12).

The first thing to do is to speak to your husband's doctor. The doctor will then be able to tell you what the various tablets are for, and also whether some tablets are more important than others. It might then be possible for you to concentrate your efforts on getting your husband to take just some of the tablets.

It is sometimes possible for a doctor to cut down on the total number of tablets that are being prescribed. Often, however, this will not be possible because the tablets are needed to treat a serious disorder, such as high blood pressure, heart failure, diabetes or epilepsy. If your husband has a general problem with swallowing, it may be possible for him to have some types of medication in liquid form.

At some point it may be necessary for you to decide how far you are prepared to go to get your husband to take medication. Some carers feel it is wrong to force or trick someone to take medication against their will. Others feel less concerned provided they believe that the person lacks the capacity to consent to treatment and are convinced that the medication is in the person's best interest.

SLEEPING

Because of my dementia I seem to have lost the 'off switch' in my brain to get to sleep. I get quite agitated in the evening and find it difficult to become calm and quiet by bedtime. What can I do? Will a sleeping pill help?

A range of practical measures can sometimes provide an effective alternative to sleeping pills. Try to establish a routine. For example, you may sleep better if you can have your main meal of the day at lunchtime, perhaps followed by a short nap, have some exercise morning and afternoon, avoid tea and coffee, keep the evenings quiet, perhaps have a warm bath and make sure your bedroom is comfortable. Some people like a night-cap: a herbal tea, warm milk or a glass of whisky.

If these measures fail to improve matters, and if your tiredness is making it difficult for you to cope, it may be necessary to consider sleeping pills. You may find, though, that these increase your confusion. (See the section 'Treating symptoms' in Chapter 12 for more information on sleeping pills.)

Some days my husband sleeps all day and then of course he is awake all night. As a result I get no sleep at all and become very irritable. What can I do?

Your husband is probably disorientated in time and does not recognise the difference between night and day. Try to establish a routine that will keep him as busy and active as possible during the daytime. (Information on activities is given in Chapter 5.) Unless you want to take advantage of a much needed break, don't let him take cat-naps. You may find that he sleeps better at night if you are able to go for daily walks together.

To help him sleep at night, make sure that he is comfortable in bed and that the room is neither too hot nor too cold. Thick curtains to cut out the light will be helpful. If he will not settle easily in a bed, he may sleep quite comfortably in a large chair or on a sofa.

Before he goes to bed at night, make sure that he uses the toilet. This will make him less likely to wake at night and will also help avoid possible bed-wetting. If he does get up during the night, try gently reminding him that it is still night-time. You might then be able to lead him quite easily back to bed. Another possibility is to distract him for a while and then suggest that it is time for you both to go to bed. Be as firm and reassuring as possible.

5 | Communication and activities

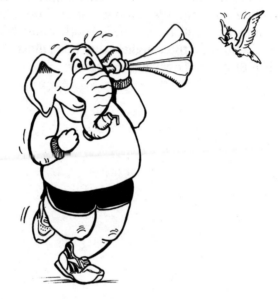

As dementia progresses, communication becomes more difficult. People with dementia develop problems both in expressing themselves clearly and in understanding what is being said to them. Communication problems can be very frustrating and upsetting for everyone concerned – for carers and people with dementia alike. This chapter aims to help you preserve the channels of communication for as long as you possibly can. Also included in this chapter are practical suggestions for helping people with dementia to make the most of their failing memories. Finally, the chapter looks at ideas for keeping people with dementia occupied, so helping them to have as enjoyable a life as possible.

IMPROVING COMMUNICATION

*My mother's dementia is getting worse and I am desperate
not to lose the ability to communicate with her. Can you
advise me?*

Communication does become increasingly difficult as dementia progresses. However, there are quite a number of things that you can do to help you and your mother to communicate:

- Make sure that she can see, hear and speak as well as possible (check hearing aids, glasses and dentures).

- Attract your mother's attention before you speak to her, perhaps by gently touching her arm.

- Try to avoid other distractions, such as from a television (tell her first that you would like to turn it off so that you can talk to her).

- While you are conversing with her, try to keep your head and shoulders at the same level as hers.

- Try to maintain eye contact when either of you is speaking (this will help keep her attention).

- Hold her hand during your conversation (another way of keeping her attention).

- Try to remain as calm as possible.

- Speak as clearly as you can.

- Use short sentences and try to talk about only one thing at a time.

- Give your mother plenty of time to answer or to show that she has understood.

- Write things down if your mother finds this helpful.

- Watch your mother's body language for visual clues as to how she might be feeling.

- Remember that you also can communicate non-verbally with your mother – for example, by your facial expressions or by giving her a hug.

My husband, who has dementia, often starts to tell me something and then is unable to go on. It is so frustrating for both of us. What can we do?

It may help your husband if he knows that he has your full attention when he is speaking, and that you understand his difficulties. You can convey this to him by maintaining eye contact throughout the conversation, and by being positive and cheerful if he loses track. He may also find it helpful if you gently nod your head from time to time to show that you are following what he is saying.

Remember that touch can often be a valuable aid to communication. Holding your husband's hand while he speaks will not only help him to maintain his concentration, it will also help to provide security in what must sometimes be for him a very baffling world. Such non-verbal communication is even more important in the later stages of dementia, when normal communication sometimes becomes impossible.

As communication with your husband becomes more difficult, it is very important for you to have your own opportunities for conversation. Friends, family members, neighbours, other carers, even the local shopkeeper can all help you with this.

My wife thinks she does all the chores, such as the cooking and shopping, and cannot accept that I now have to do everything. How can I explain this to her?

Your wife may no longer be able to remember what she has just done. However, she can remember doing household chores on many previous occasions, and these are what she is remembering now. There really is no point in trying to explain the situation to her. She will not be able to acknowledge or thank you for all the extra work you are doing. It may help you to feel better if you can sometimes remind yourself that without your devotion and care it would not be possible for your wife to continue to live at home.

MEMORY AIDS

I have been diagnosed with Alzheimer's disease. Does exercising the brain slow down the progress of dementia?

There is no clear answer to this question, but mental activity – such as reading, playing games, painting, etc. – may help. But don't overdo it. Make sure that your 'brain gym' is achievable and enjoyable. (See also the section 'Activities' later in this chapter).

My wife is in the very early stages of Alzheimer's disease and is frustrated by her loss of memory. What can I do to help her?

A useful way of helping your wife cope with her loss of memory is to encourage her to make the most of everyday memory aids and also to devise personalised 'memory joggers'. We all rely on information given by clocks, calendars, diaries, newspapers and so on. People with memory problems need these everyday aids all the more. They will also find it easier to manage if they can have their own memory joggers, such as message boards, handy lists and instruction sheets.

It will probably be best if you and your wife can work together to devise a range of memory aids that suit her needs. However, here are few points you might like to consider:

- Keep familiar objects in their usual places, where your wife can see them easily.

- Make sure that watches and clocks show the correct time.

- Indicate today's date on any calendars, perhaps by marking off the days as they pass.

- Put up a message board in a prominent place and establish a habit of using it.

- Make a list of the day's activities and put it somewhere that it can be found easily. Encourage your wife to refer to it often and to tick off each activity as it is completed.

- If she has to be left alone at home, leave a clear note saying where you are and when you are due back. Try to establish a regular pattern so that your absences are part of a routine.

- Put up photographs of family members and close friends, all clearly named. Or add names to pictures in an album and encourage her to look at them often.

- People in the early stages of Alzheimer's disease often have their own ways to aid their memory.

I get so frustrated because my wife forgets things that have just happened. Is it possible to re-train the memory of someone with Alzheimer's disease?

One of the main problems with Alzheimer's disease is the failure of short-term memory. This means that people forget things that have just happened. If you think about it, without looking at your watch, you could have a fairly good guess as to what time of day it is. You would also probably be able to remember when you last had a drink, what you had for breakfast and what month of the year it is. Such things tend to get lost in Alzheimer's disease, and people become confused as a result. For example, they may forget that they have just eaten lunch and ask for lunch again.

Most people think it is not possible to re-train the memory of someone with Alzheimer's disease. It may, however, be possible to help them to devise memory aids and joggers to help them function better, at least in the early stages of the illness. For example, a person with Alzheimer's disease might be able to continue to make a cup of tea if he or she has the instructions for doing this written down on a card. It would, however, still be necessary for the person to remember to look at the card and to be able to follow the steps one by one.

Some people find message boards and scribble pads useful in the early stages of the illness. (See also the previous answer for more memory-jogging ideas.) The Alzheimer's Society publishes a booklet for people with dementia, called *I'm told I have Dementia.*

My wife has Alzheimer's disease. Is it a good thing to keep going over the events of the day with her to try to help her remember them? Or is this just a waste of time?

Even if you go over them with her, your wife might not be able to remember things that she has just done or that have just been said. This loss of short-term memory is one of the main symptoms of Alzheimer's disease. If you want to help your wife recall things, the best strategy is to use statements rather than questions. Instead of 'Do you remember . . .' talk about the events of the day. This will help you wife have some sense of what has happened and of time passing. The best thing to do is to try to enjoy things together at the time of doing them.

ACTIVITIES

My husband is in the early stages of Alzheimer's disease. Have you any suggestions for the kind of things he could be doing?

In the earlier stages of the condition, it will not be too difficult for your husband to be occupied. He will probably be happy to help you with everyday household tasks, such as dusting and polishing, and laying and clearing the table. It does not really matter if he forgets what he has done and does these things again and again. He may also be able to help you with preparing food and doing the washing up. If you have a garden, this can present plenty of opportunities for simple activities.

A daily walk will probably do you both good and will also provide topics of conversation. If you keep an eye on him, he is likely to be able to go with you to the local shops. If he has been used to going to the pub or eating out, it is a good idea to help him to continue to do so for as long as he can.

In some areas (contact your local branch of the Alzheimer's Society) there may be support groups for people with dementia, or 'Alzheimer Cafés' where people meet to socialise. It might also be a good idea for your husband to go to a day centre (see later in this section and also the section 'Day care' in Chapter 9).

Assuming that he is fairly sociable, your husband will probably enjoy having friends and relatives to visit him at home. Generally, it is best to avoid large gatherings as these will be more difficult for him to cope with. If possible, warn any prospective visitors beforehand if they are not already aware of your husband's problems with his memory.

While your husband is still in the early stages of the illness, it would be a good idea to help him to prepare a scrapbook of his life, containing photographs and other souvenirs of earlier days. This will help him to remember his past for longer as the disease progresses. It could also be useful later on for strangers who may be helping to look after him. They will be able to go over the scrapbook with him.

Keeping your husband occupied in the later stages of the illness will be more of a problem, but it is worth making the effort. This will not only help him to get the most from life but will also help prevent other health problems – such as those that might arise from lack of exercise. Gentle exercises, such as moving to music, are often very popular. Repetitive tasks, perhaps based on previous interests, can be useful for maintaining interest and passing the time. Your husband may like being read to, and also listening to music – even if he wants the same piece over and over again!

My husband still enjoys going out on his own and finding his way home. However, he always goes to the same shop – a local optician's. He stands at the counter and makes conversation. Eventually he leaves but he seems to have developed a fixation on this particular shop. What can I do about it?

This sounds to be a fairly harmless activity. It is probably best to explain to the shop assistant what your husband's problem is and suggest that they find ways of reassuring him and gently telling him to go back home. If you are worried about your husband getting lost, you might consider getting him to carry some form of identification (see also the section 'Wandering' in Chapter 6).

My mother has been diagnosed with Alzheimer's disease but is still living on her own with her two cats. She is very attached to them. Do you think it will be all right for her to keep them?

Keeping animals may be beneficial to some people with Alzheimer's disease, especially in the early stage of the illness. Animals provide companionship and help keep people active. As long as you feel that you mother is able to care properly for her cats, it would be best to leave them where they are. If you think she is not coping, it would be best to make other arrangements. If you or one of your mother's neighbours could take the cats, your mother would still be able to see them. If this is not possible, discuss the problem with the local Cats Protection League or RSPCA.

It has been suggested that my wife should start going to a day centre. What sort of activities will there be at the centre for someone with Alzheimer's disease?

Day centres vary, but a variety of activities will probably take place. What exactly happens depends on how many people attend, how severe their dementia is and how well trained the staff are.

Practical help given at a day centre may include bathing, hairdressing and chiropody. Lunch is provided. Other activities, often done in groups, may include listening to music, doing simple exercises and reminiscence therapy (see the section 'Psychological treatments' in Chapter 12). Sometimes outings to shops and to local places of interest may be organised. (See also the section 'Day care' in Chapter 9 for more information about day centres.)

HOLIDAYS

My husband and I always enjoyed our holidays together. He now has dementia and is probably getting too confused to go on an ordinary holiday but is there any way we could go away together? I could really do with a holiday myself.

There are many kinds of holiday venues that cater for people with different disabilities and which will make you and your husband welcome. They range from private guest houses to well-equipped specialist holiday centres. If you choose the right one you will find that people are sympathetic and understanding of your difficulties.

Many Alzheimer's Society branches organise group holidays and many arrange day trips for people with dementia and their carers. The Alzheimer's Society also has an arrangement with Vitalise, a charity (formerly called Winged Fellowship Trust) that provides holidays for people with disabilities. Special weeks are set aside in their special holiday centres to take people with dementia and their carers. Contact Vitalise to find out more (address in Appendix 1).

Alzheimer Scotland may also be able to help with holidays. (See Appendix 1 for the contact details of relevant organisations.)

I am planning a holiday and have just been diagnosed with Alzheimer's disease. Do I need to mention this to the insurance company?

Yes, you must tell them or the insurance will not be valid. If you were to fall ill while on the holiday, the company might refuse to pay out. RADAR (contact details in Appendix 1) can provide information about companies that specialise in holiday insurance for people with disabilities.

It is possible some companies might refuse to insure you. Others will consider cases individually but may charge a higher rate. So do shop around.

We have been planning a holiday for some time now to visit our son and his young family in Australia. However, my wife has just been diagnosed with Alzheimer's disease. Do you think we should still go?

As your wife has only recently been diagnosed, she should still be able to make this trip. A trip to see family members can be very important. However, it would be wise to seek advice from the doctor, as your wife's ability to cope with the trip will depend on her particular condition.

People with even mild dementia may find long-haul travel especially difficult. In addition to the journey itself and subsequent jet-lag, your wife may be disorientated by the new environment. You may want to break the journey with a stop-over.

If you do decide to go, you will need to take advice about travel insurance for your wife (see the previous answer).

6 | Personal safety

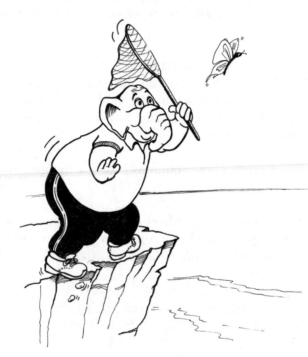

Questions on topics relating to the personal safety of people with dementia become increasingly important as the disease progresses. This chapter draws attention to a range of commonly encountered risks, both inside and outside the home. It offers carers useful advice on how they might help to reduce the risk of accidents while still allowing the people they care for to have as much independence as possible. It is important to balance risks with depriving someone of their independence.

LIVING ALONE

My father shows signs of increasing confusion. How can I tell when it's no longer safe for him to live alone?

It is difficult to make a hard-and-fast rule. Many confused people do survive on their own for years in apparently hazardous conditions. They can even be helped to do so by a common-sense appraisal of the surroundings and the removal of the most obvious dangers. There are, however, a number of key pointers to a person's inability to continue living alone. You should take account of the following warning signs:

- carelessness about fire hazards (gas fires are the worst);

- leaving his home, particularly at night, and failing to find the way back;

- repeated complaints and expressions of anxiety by neighbours who were previously tolerant and helpful;

- a state of squalor that is inconsistent with the confused person's previous personality and personal dignity.

People have a right to live in their own home if at all possible and you should try to help your father to do so if he wants to (see Chapter 9 for information on getting help). A range of electronic and computer-assisted devices has been developed to help people with memory problems to cope with various aspects of home management. Ask the Alzheimer's Society (contact details in Appendix 1) for advice.

DANGERS AT HOME

My mother still prefers to live on her own even though she has dementia. I am particularly worried that she will have an accident with the gas. What can I do?

Gas suppliers keep a register of customers who need special attention and special services. If your mother is not already on such a register, you should contact her gas supplier. It is also worth noting that free gas-safety checks are available to people living alone who are registered disabled, receiving Disability Benefit or over 60 years old. If the gas safety of your mother's home has not been checked recently, you should arrange a check as soon as possible. It will probably be useful if you can be present when the check is carried out. This will be reassuring for your mother and will give you the opportunity to ask questions if you need more information.

If your mother is in the habit of turning on gas taps without lighting the gas, you should have the gas disconnected. She would probably then be dependent on someone else to do her cooking for her. If your mother is going to continue using gas, it might be useful to ask her gas supplier to fit a gas detector. However, such a device will be of use only if your mother is able to respond appropriately if it goes off.

My elderly aunt with dementia still lives alone, with morning and evening visits from care workers. Sometimes she forgets to turn the lights off and I'm worried she will leave an electric fire on and cause a fire. Is there anything I can do?

If the wiring and electrical appliances in your aunt's home are not new, you may wish to have them checked by a qualified electrician. Sometimes electricity suppliers will do this free.

You might also advise her to use one of the safer forms of electric heating. For example, modern fan heaters and oil-filled electric radiators are both generally safer than radiant bar electric fires. Also, a circuit breaker between an electrical appliance and the electricity socket will provide added safety. If your aunt has central heating, it might be better to get rid of electric fires altogether.

Time switches would provide a simple means of ensuring that your aunt's lights and electrical appliances are turned on and off at appropriate times. It would also be a good idea to tell the electricity supplier of your aunt's special needs. Electricity suppliers should keep a register of older customers and those at possible risk.

My father, who has Alzheimer's disease and now lives with us, is a smoker. I worry about the possibility of fire. How can I stop him smoking?

The chances are that as your father's illness progresses he will forget about smoking. You may be able to bring this time forward if you remove his cigarettes and then don't do anything to remind him about smoking. If you smoke yourself, you should probably also stop or at least go and smoke somewhere that he cannot see you.

If your father becomes very agitated when you remove his cigarettes, it is probably wisest to let him continue smoking for a while before repeating your withdrawal tactic. You could meanwhile try to encourage him to cut down on the number of cigarettes he smokes and get him to try nicotine patches (which can sometimes be obtained free from the NHS). As long as he continues to smoke, you and other people who care for him will need to try to supervise him whenever he has a cigarette. Make sure his clothes and furniture are fire-resistant and that waste-paper bins are not near where he sits. Rather than matches, make sure he has a lighter that doesn't continue to burn after he has put it down. A smoke alarm is always a good idea.

My wife has fallen several times in the house recently. Can you suggest how I might reduce the risk of falls?

Trying to make the home as hazard-free as possible makes good sense for everyone. It is particularly important when a person's risk of falling is increased by old age or confusion. Some common hazards that should be dealt with include:

- loose or torn carpets, especially on the stairs or in doorways;
- loose mats;
- highly polished floors;
- broken or loose stair rods;
- inadequate rails on the stairs;
- poor lighting (it would be worth having night-lights if your wife often gets up at night);
- trailing electric flexes;
- wobbly or damaged furniture;
- furniture with protruding legs;
- clutter, such as shoes or newspapers, left on the floor;
- lack of or inadequate safety measures in the bathroom;
- worn slippers or other footwear that may cause tripping.

If you think you need further help, your wife's doctor or someone from Social Services will probably be able to arrange for an occupational therapist to come and advise you.

My husband has had a number of quite bad falls. So far our son has always been around to help, but I am 85 and would not be able to lift my husband on my own. What should I do if he falls when we are alone?

If your husband falls and is in pain, the best thing to do is to cover him with a blanket, give him a pillow if he can move his head freely, reassure him and tell him that you are going to get help. Then either telephone the doctor if the fall seems serious or seek help from someone nearby.

If your husband appears to be unhurt, try putting a chair beside him and then encouraging him to use the chair to try to get up while you give him as much help as you can. If he can't understand what to do or if he is unable to get up when he tries, make him comfortable and then seek help.

WANDERING

My father, who has Alzheimer's, still likes to go for short walks on his own. I am worried that he will get lost and come to harm. What precautions can I take?

If your father's walks take him out for only a short while, and he is currently returning without much difficulty, there is probably not too much cause for concern. Indeed, the exercise he gets should be beneficial to both of you – and he is less likely to be restless when at home.

It would be sensible to make sure that your father always has his name, address and phone number on him. Alzheimer Scotland and the Alzheimer's Society have produced cards that a person with dementia can carry. You may wish to purchase a special Medic-Alert bracelet or SOS talisman (contact details for these companies are in Appendix 1) bearing the essential contact information.

Alternatively, you could have a bracelet tag engraved at a local jewellers.

Another precaution would be to inform your local police station that your father has problems with his memory and his sense of time and place. Similarly, it is advisable to make sure that neighbours, the local shops and any other likely destinations are aware of the problem.

You should prepare yourself for the likely decline in your father's memory, which may cause him to get temporarily lost. It is very worrying when someone goes missing. If they do, alert the neighbours and also the police.

My wife has been wandering out of the house and has once done this at night. My family keep telling me that I should ask the doctor for some medication. Can you advise?

It is best to avoid medication because the amount needed may produce undesirable side effects, such as drowsiness, falls and incontinence (for more about sleeping pills, see the section 'Treating symptoms' in Chapter 12). It is better to make your home as secure as possible, ideally fitting bolts to the tops and bottoms of all outer doors.

My husband keeps wandering out of the house and getting lost. I feel so guilty when he keeps being brought back by the police. Why does he do this?

No one can be expected to keep a 24-hour watch on someone else, so you should not blame yourself or others who have been left in charge of your husband. Wandering is quite common in people with dementia.

There are various possible reasons why your husband may be wandering. If he has always been an active person, it may simply be that he has excess energy which he needs to use up. Alternatively, he may be wandering to relieve boredom caused by poor concentration (see Chapter 5 for ideas about how he could be occupied). A further possibility is that he may be looking for someone or something in his past which he just cannot remember.

My wife has wandered off and got lost several times. She has always come back home or been brought back, but I never know what to do. Can you advise?

Although it is very worrying when people with dementia get lost, they are not likely to come to any harm. The risk to your wife will obviously vary depending on where she gets lost.

As a general piece of advice, the best thing you can do if your wife goes missing is to try to remain calm and not panic. A first step might be to check the various places where your wife is known, such as your local shops. You should tell neighbours and friends.

It is generally best to contact the police sooner rather than later. To help the police and other searchers, it would be a good idea to keep a recent photograph of your wife close at hand and also to be able to give a clear description of the clothes she is wearing. It would also be worth persuading her to wear some sort of identification, as discussed in the first answer in this section.

DRIVING

Is it true that people with dementia can drive a car?

Research suggests that many people with dementia continue to drive after the onset of the illness, but in an unsafe fashion. However, a small number of people with dementia seem to preserve their driving ability for a while. This is possibly associated with the fact that people in the early stages of dementia may still retain the ability to do things that they learned earlier on in their lives.

The main problem is that, as dementia progresses, so the ability to drive inevitably deteriorates, but usually without the affected person realising that this is happening. It is very important that anyone who has become an unsafe driver should not be allowed to continue driving, however upsetting this may be. The key is regular assessment and review.

How can I persuade my husband, who has dementia, that he is no longer safe to drive a car?

Some people with Alzheimer's disease realise that they are no longer safe and give up driving easily. However, many others, like your husband, have no understanding that their skills are diminishing and that they no longer have the usual reactions or memory for driving. This can be an extremely difficult problem to manage.

If you don't need to use the car yourself, you should consider selling it so that your husband is not constantly reminded of it. If you want to continue driving the car, one possibility would be to make it difficult for your husband to find the car keys and then find ways of distracting him whenever he suggests driving. If you go out together in the car, you could suggest that you need the driving practice as you are a less experienced driver than he is.

Anyone affected by a medical condition that impairs their ability to drive is legally bound to inform the DVLA (contact details in Appendix 1). If your husband is unable or unwilling to do this, you or his doctor should inform the DVLA on his behalf. The DVLA may offer a repeat driving test if necessary. You should also inform your car insurance company about your husband's diagnosis.

After your husband has stopped driving, you may be able to help him to retain his sense of independence if you suggest that he organises a taxi or mini-cab account.

I have been told I have dementia. Can I still drive a car?

Diagnosis of dementia is not in itself a reason to stop driving. You will eventually have to stop but many people continue to drive safely for some time after the diagnosis. However, you may not be able to judge when you become unsafe and you must ask a trusted person to tell you and make sure you stop. You must inform the DVLA and your car insurance company (see above). There's a lot to be said for walking!

7 | Behaviour that may cause difficulties

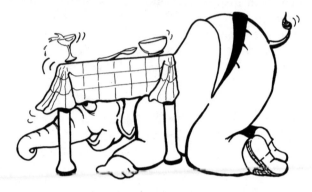

Alzheimer's disease and other dementias sometimes cause people to behave in ways that are difficult for others to live with. For example, people with dementia may become restless or aggressive for no obvious reason. It is important to remember that their behaviour is affected by their illness and that they are probably not behaving badly on purpose. Remember, too, that their capabilities and their behaviour can fluctuate from day to day and even during different times of the day. This chapter gives suggestions for managing some of the more common difficulties.

ANNOYING BEHAVIOUR

Sometimes my wife does very silly things and then looks at me blankly. I get the feeling that she is being deliberately annoying. Can this be the case?

It is very unlikely that this is the case. Most people who have looked after someone with dementia have at some time or another felt that they are being taken for a ride or that the other person is being deliberately mischievous. People with dementia often do child-like things or may just appear bewildered or perplexed at times. This is a result of the illness. It is not a deliberate attempt to annoy.

As your wife's dementia advances, her difficult behaviour may make you feel increasingly bitter and angry. Don't feel guilty about these feelings. They are extremely common and understandable. If you discuss this with your local carers' group, you will be surprised how many other people feel the same way.

My husband keeps on asking me the same question over and over again. How can I learn to be patient?

Your husband keeps asking the same question over and over because he forgets the answer, then also forgets the question he asked.

Sometimes, instead of answering the question for the umpteenth time, tell your husband that everything is fine and that you are taking care of things. Try to make him feel more secure. It might also help if you write the answer down. If he asks you the question again, you can then direct him to the written answer instead of answering the question yourself.

If your husband continues to ask one particular question, despite answers and reassurances, try to distract him by changing the subject or hugging him. Also, when he is not asking the question, give him lots of love and affection. Eventually (and it may be a while) he may stop asking it.

LOSING THINGS

My mother, who has dementia but still lives on her own, keeps losing her cheque book. However, I always find it somewhere, usually hidden under a cushion or under the bed but well out of sight. What can be done?

Because your mother has dementia, it is inevitable that she will lose things. Eventually you might need to take charge of her cheque book and other important documents yourself. In the meantime, you will probably discover her favourite hiding places. Encourage her to look there first.

My father sometimes loses his keys and locks himself out of his flat. He wants to carry on living on his own although he has Alzheimer's disease. What can I do?

It would be a good idea to make several copies of your father's keys. You could then put one set in a safe place in your father's flat, keep one set yourself and ideally give a set to a helpful neighbour. Don't put your father's name and address on his keys in case a potential thief picks them up.

My mother frequently loses things and then accuses me and her 'home help' (home care assistant) of stealing them. How should we respond to, and deal with, these accusations?

Generally, you should try not to take these accusations too seriously. Your mother's loss of memory increases the chance that she will misplace things. Because her things often go 'missing', she may well create her own safe hiding places for them. Unfortunately, she will also forget where these hiding places are, thus making the problem even worse.

It is usually pointless to contradict accusations of this type. You risk getting drawn into an argument with your mother, which may make her more upset. It is best to try searching for the object in question and to reassure her that you know where the missing item is. Try to discover any regular hiding places that she may have. Keep replacements of important items, such as spectacles and keys. Try to get into the habit of checking waste-bins before emptying them.

Try to make sure that your mother's 'home help', friends and neighbours understand the reason for your mother's behaviour so that they don't get upset.

It is worth bearing in mind that, occasionally, when a person with dementia makes an accusation of theft, there may be some substance in it. If your mother's accusations involve money, you should investigate as thoroughly as possible. Try to minimise her need to have cash or valuables in the house, thus reducing any opportunity for theft by outsiders.

Depending on your mother's personality, you may have to prepare yourself for an increase in such accusations. Some people seem to be naturally more suspicious than others, and such personality traits may be exaggerated by dementia. Sometimes medication may help with this problem. Your GP will advise you as necessary.

NON-RECOGNITION

Sometimes, in the evenings, my husband looks at me and asks me when I am leaving. He then hands me the telephone and says 'Tell my wife to come home, so that you can go back to your home'. What can I do?

This can be a very distressing occurrence. This behaviour relates to your husband's poor memory and his inability to recognise you. He is remembering you as you were in the earlier part of his life. The best thing you can do in this situation is to give him a hug and remind him who you are. Then try to distract him, perhaps with a walk to the kitchen to make a cup of tea or some other activity that you can enjoy together.

My wife often says to me 'When are you going to take me home?' Then she packs some things into a bag – pictures, ornaments, etc. How can I explain that this is her home?

Home can mean so many things. It might mean the childhood home that your wife may still remember as a place of safety, warmth and familiarity. People with dementia can find it difficult to relate to their surroundings. When they look around they may not recognise anything and this may make them feel very insecure or upset.

You need to give your wife lots of hugs and reassurance. Ask her to talk about her home, and reassure her that all is well and that you are looking after her. It is best not to enter into any sort of argument with her. If she is convinced that she is not at home, you could try taking her out on a short walk with her bag and then return home and help her to unpack.

HALLUCINATIONS

My mother, who has Alzheimer's disease, seems to be having hallucinations. She holds conversations when there is no one there to talk to and seems to see things that don't exist. Sometimes she becomes very frightened and upset. How should I respond?

Hallucinations – in which people see, hear or sense the presence of someone or something that is not there – are quite a common symptom in Alzheimer's disease and Lewy body dementia. It is not surprising that your mother sometimes becomes frightened and upset because hallucinations can seem very real.

If your mother becomes distressed by a hallucination, offer her reassurance and physical comfort by giving her a hug or holding her hand. Do not pretend that the content of her hallucination is real, but also do not get into any arguments about this. Keep as calm as possible and try gently to distract her, perhaps by offering her a drink or drawing her attention to something else in the room. Fortunately, even recurrent hallucinations usually last only a few days or weeks and then are forgotten.

Hallucinations are sometimes associated with poor vision, so it would be worth getting your mother's eyes tested. Also, if rooms are well lit she may be less likely to misinterpret what she is seeing.

It would also be wise to talk to your mother's doctor, particularly if she has Lewy body dementia, which requires specialist advice. Medical treatment is sometimes helpful (discussed in the section 'Drug treatment' in Chapter 12), or it may be necessary to adjust other medications that can cause hallucinations as a side effect.

RESTLESSNESS AND AGITATION

My husband, who has Alzheimer's, gets sudden bouts of restlessness. Why is this, and how should I manage?

Restlessness is a very common feature of Alzheimer's disease. It can make the affected person very agitated, and sometimes leads to wandering (discussed in Chapter 6). Restlessness has a number of possible causes, some of which can be avoided.

If restlessness comes on suddenly, it may be due to pain or discomfort. Toothache is a common cause of pain, which should always be investigated and treated. Digestive problems, such as indigestion and constipation, also commonly cause pain or discomfort, but can often be avoided if attention is paid to the diet (see the section 'Food and drink' in Chapter 4). Discomfort due to a full bladder is an extremely common cause of restlessness, so it is worth ensuring that your husband visits the toilet frequently. If he has difficulty passing urine, he may have a urinary tract infection that needs medical attention.

Almost any drug your husband is taking could cause restlessness. You should therefore check with his doctor to see if any of his medications might be reduced or stopped. Caffeinated drinks, such as tea or coffee, can also cause or aggravate restlessness and agitation.

Another possibility is that your husband's restlessness is due to boredom, in which case it might help if you can find more activities for him (see Chapter 5 for ideas). Sudden bouts of restlessness can often be relieved by going out for a walk or taking some other form of exercise.

If none of these suggestions works, it might mean that your husband is feeling anxious and upset. In which case, it might help him if you give him hugs or sit with him for a while, perhaps holding his hand or reading to him.

I get very agitated in the evening, like a wound-up clockwork toy. How can my sister, who looks after me, help me to calm down?

You could both ensure that there is an established routine of quiet in the late afternoon, avoiding caffeine and sitting calmly. Your sister needs to make sure that you have no worries on your mind in the evening, and that she gives you the impression she has everything under control.

My elderly mother, who has dementia and lives with us, sometimes has screaming fits. Why is this and what can I do about it?

People with dementia often have a phase of screaming fits. The first thing you should do is to ask your mother's doctor to check for any possible physical reason for the screaming, such as pain or constipation. It may help the doctor if you notice whether there is any pattern to the screaming; for example, is it just around mealtimes?

If no physical cause is found, it is probable that your mother just feels bewildered. Try to keep calm, hold her often and make her feel loved and supported. If the screaming persists, she may need a small amount of sedation from the doctor, as well as plenty of comfort from you. Usually this distressing phase passes and the sedation can be stopped.

ANGER AND AGGRESSION

When I try to explain to my wife that she has done or said something wrong, she becomes very defensive and angry and blames me and tells me to leave. I find this very upsetting. What can I do?

It is not surprising that you find this upsetting. However, you must remind yourself that your wife's problems are due to the disease. She cannot help it when she does or says something wrong. Having made the mistake, she may either want to conceal it or have no recollection at all of what she has done. In either case, it would be best for you to try to avoid drawing attention to your wife's failures and to keep as calm as you can. Any type of conflict is likely to cause distress both for you and for your wife.

I have dementia and I tend to follow my husband around, and need to know what he's doing all the time. Sometimes I get frustrated and I swear and shout and say awful things to him. How can I stop doing this?

Following someone around is quite normal. Your husband needs to understand you are trying your best to cope. It sounds as if you want him to read your mind and reassure you all the time. Obviously, this is not possible, but you can both try to talk openly about this and do your best to communicate and listen to each other. Perhaps your husband can make sure you know what he is doing, and leave you a note if he goes anywhere.

Sometimes I think my father must really hate me. He has Alzheimer's disease and I have moved in with him. I want to carry on caring for him but he gets so angry with me and says such awful things. What might I be doing wrong?

Although it is natural for you to blame yourself, it is very important for you to understand that your father's anger is not really aimed at you. You are not causing his anger. The anger is part of his illness. It is common for people who have Alzheimer's disease to pass through a phase of being angry and sometimes aggressive.

Although this angry phase will pass, it may help you in the meantime to consider some of the things that may be triggering your father's anger. A community mental health nurse (see the section 'Services for people at home' in Chapter 9) could visit your home to help you with this.

There are many possible reasons why your father may be feeling so angry. For example, he may not like being forced to accept help to do things that he used to do on his own, such as washing. Or perhaps he feels frustrated simply because he is unable to do certain things. Another possibility is that your father is bewildered and frightened because he no longer understands what is going on around him. It is also possible that he is just bored or has an excess of energy. Sometimes, hunger, the need to pass urine or constipation can lead to disruptive behaviour. If the angry outbursts have started only recently, they may be due to an infection or pain. Once you have been able to identify some of the things that tend to make your father angry, you may be able to reduce the number of his angry outbursts.

My husband, who has dementia, often gets angry and sometimes hits me. He never used to do this. What can I do to calm things down?

It is important to remember that your husband's anger is not aimed directly at you – it is part of his illness (see the previous answer). You may find that you get very angry yourself and even want to hit him back. However, this is quite likely to make the situation worse. When this happens, try to react calmly. If you can manage to distract him, he will probably forget quite quickly why he has been so angry. If you feel you are in any danger, it would be wise to leave the room for a while. You might also call a friend or neighbour. If you do feel that you are in danger, you must consider your own safety and your husband's long-term interests, and inform Social Services.

In certain circumstances, drugs may help to calm your husband down. You should talk to your husband's doctor about the benefits and drawbacks of the tranquillisers that are available (see the section 'Treating symptoms' in Chapter 12).

Above all, try not to get disheartened or frustrated with the care you are giving your husband. This distressing phase always passes after a time. When your husband is calm, give him plenty of love and affection.

My mother has dementia. She never used to swear but now she seems to swear all the time. It doesn't matter who is present. What should I do?

You are probably surprised that your mother even knows the words that she uses! The fact is that most of us know these words but would not usually bring them into our conversation. The normal brain has an inbuilt mechanism that tells us the difference between appropriate and inappropriate behaviour and language. When certain areas of the brain are affected by dementia or another disease, this mechanism is impaired. Swearing may be the only way in which your mother can express anger, anxiety, discomfort or pain.

You may find it useful to ask a community mental health nurse (see the section 'Services for people at home' in Chapter 9) or other health professional to help you to find out whether there are any particular situations that appear to trigger your mother's bad language. You might then be able to help her to avoid these situations.

SEXUAL BEHAVIOUR

Is it common for people with dementia to show unusual sexual behaviour?

People with dementia, both men and women, do sometimes display inappropriate sexual behaviour, although this is not common. Such behaviour may include undressing in public, fondling the genitals or touching someone in an inappropriate way. The best way to respond is to try not to over-react and to remember that the behaviour is due to the disease. Then calmly and quietly try to distract the person and encourage some other activity.

My husband, who has Alzheimer's disease, wants to have sex with me much more than he used to. I can't cope with his excessive demands for sex and am finding it all very distressing. Sometimes I want to react by sleeping in a separate bed. What should I do?

It is very understandable that you feel upset. You may feel better if you are able to remember that your husband's changed sexual behaviour is part of his illness. Your husband probably does not remember that he has just had sex with you and this is why he wants to start again.

If your husband gets angry when you refuse him, you will probably find it best to keep out of his way until the moment has passed for him or he goes to sleep. This might mean going to sleep in a separate bed sometimes. Whether or not you want to sleep separately on a permanent basis is a more difficult decision. You will probably find it helpful to talk to someone who has been trained to help people to cope with sexual problems. People who might be able to help are your community mental health nurse (formerly called community psychiatric nurse or CPN), a counsellor specialising in sexual problems or Relate (contact details in Appendix 1).

OTHER PEOPLE'S ATTITUDES

We live in a flat and my husband, who has dementia, sometimes gets noisy and disturbing, especially at night. I feel so embarrassed and ashamed. What should I tell our neighbours?

It might take some courage, but you will find it easier to manage in the long run if you apologise to your neighbours but also tell them that your husband has dementia and that he cannot help sometimes making a noise. If your neighbours have never heard of dementia, you may need to explain that it is a physical disorder of the brain that affects a person's memory, language and understanding.

My father, who has dementia, now lives with us and I am pleased to be able to care for him. However, my nine-year-old son no longer brings his friends home because he is embarrassed by his grandfather's behaviour. I am very sad about this. What can I do?

You should talk to your son about this. It is important that children realise that illnesses such as dementia are part of life – they need to be able to talk about it, both with parents and with teachers.

Encourage your son to tell his friends about his grandfather's illness. With your support, he might be able to bring his friends home, introduce them to his grandfather and then perhaps go off to his room to play. There are a number of children's books, suitable for different ages, about dementia (see Appendix 2). The Alzheimer's Society also produces a leaflet for teenagers on this subject.

I have a diagnosis of dementia. What should I say to other people?

You may find this hard to talk about, but other people can be a real help and support to you if they understand your difficulties. Perhaps you could start off by telling them you have memory problems and are likely to get worse. You may want to tell people what they can do to make your life easier, or what you don't find helpful. For example, you may not like people doing things for you.

8 | Carers' emotions

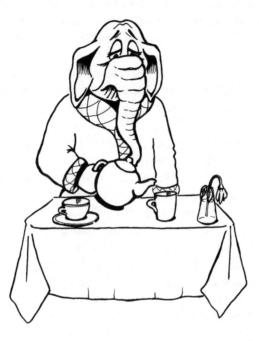

Caring for someone with dementia can be rewarding but also difficult. You may have health problems of your own. You may be tired from lack of sleep or from the constant need to pay attention to someone else. You may have worries from financial problems or about how long you can cope. You may just want a break. Your needs are just as important as the needs of the person you care for. You have a right to health and rest, to time for yourself and to stop caring if you want to. You will be able to care better for someone else if you also care for yourself.

EMOTIONAL SUPPORT

Since my wife became ill, most of our friends have stopped visiting. How can we persuade people that Alzheimer's disease is not catching and that my wife and I need friends and visitors?

It's an old cliché that in times of trouble you find out who your real friends are. But your friends probably haven't stopped liking or caring for you. It's just that they don't know how to react to the change in your lives.

Try speaking directly to the people who have been closest to your wife and yourself. Phone them or go round to see them and explain about the illness. Let them know that you haven't changed and that you and your wife need company even more. If they are real friends, they will support both you and your wife.

As a carer you certainly need all the friends you can get. Try to get breaks from caring to keep up with your old social life – going to the pub, playing golf, going to the pictures, whatever you used to enjoy doing. You need to keep space and time for your own interests and activities.

Many carers find that they make new friends if they join a carers' support group or Alzheimer's Society branch. Certainly there will be people there who understand your need for company. In some places there are visiting schemes where a volunteer will come and visit you and your wife on a regular basis. Your local library might have information on such organisations in your area, or ask Social Services for advice.

Sometimes I feel so alone. As though there is only me and my husband in the whole world. He has dementia. I don't need help. I just need someone to talk to. What can I do?

Having someone to talk to can be a great help for carers. Many people find that it is much easier to cope if they are able to share their feelings and experiences.

There are a number of different ways that you can contact people who will listen and understand. The Alzheimer's Society and Alzheimer Scotland both have telephone helplines (contact details in Appendix 1), and they can put you in touch with a local group.

In some areas there are befriending schemes that will arrange for someone to visit you in your own home. If you want to get out of the house, you will probably be able to find a carers' group that meets regularly somewhere not far from where you live. Such groups have been set up by many voluntary organisations and also by Social Services.

I'm a gay man and I care for my partner of twenty years who has dementia. I go to a carers' group but I don't feel very welcome. It's not that they are unkind but I know they don't think my relationship is the same as theirs or my pain as real. Is there anywhere I can get help from people who really understand?

Some carers' groups are better than others at making people welcome. It's a pity that the one you went to didn't help you, as your experience of caring is the same as anyone else's and your feelings are just as important.

Many cities now have groups for gay carers. Most of them focus on caring for people with AIDS, some of whom develop dementia. You may find that one of these groups is relevant to your needs. Ring your local gay helpline to find out about carers' groups in your area, or contact the Terrence Higgins Trust (contact details in Appendix 1).

The national Alzheimer's Society (contact details in Appendix 1) has a confidential gay carers' network.

LOSS AND DESPAIR

Sometimes I feel such a terrible sense of loss and despair now that my husband has Alzheimer's disease. It makes me just want to sit down and give up. How can I get help for my feelings?

You first started to help yourself when you admitted how over-whelming these feelings are. As Alzheimer's disease progresses, you may feel sometimes that the illness is robbing you of the person you used to know. You may feel a great loss of companionship. In many ways it is like grieving for the death of someone who is still alive.

Grief is common among people like you who are caring for some-one with a long-term illness. You may find yourself shifting between hope and despair, thinking your husband may get better and then knowing that he won't.

Don't be afraid of these feelings. They are real and natural. Try to focus on the small things you can do to make life as pleasant as pos-sible for your husband, and look for the parts of his personality that are still there.

It always helps to find someone to talk to. Share your feelings with family and friends, join a carers' group or talk to your social worker, community mental health nurse, or someone in your local Alzheimer's Society Branch.

My father has had Alzheimer's for six years. He is very restless and nearly always distressed. He searches the house endlessly looking for my mother who has been dead for four years. He cries a lot. I just cannot find a way of comforting him. At night when he's asleep I think I could just smother him with the pillow and it would be better for both of us. I know that's not true but I'm scared I might do it. What can I do?

Such feelings are common. Dementia brings a terrible sense of loss to all of those involved. You feel a deep loss for your father as a person who once cared for you, he feels his whole life slipping away from him and longs for the security of the past as represented by his wife. It's very painful to see the distress of another person and be unable to help.

You must talk to someone about your feelings, perhaps a close member of the family, a friend or the Alzheimer's Society or Alzheimer Scotland helpline.The Samaritans provide a confidential 24-hour helpline (see Appendix 1).

Your feelings and your fears are nothing to be ashamed of. Try to get more breaks from caring; involve other family members. Talk to your doctor or social worker about how you can reduce your father's anxiety. Make sure they know how hard you are finding things and insist on having proper support and respite breaks (see the section 'Respite care' in Chapter 9). You should not have to take on this burden alone.

ANGER AND BITTERNESS

Is it normal to get angry and lose my temper when my mother repeats things endlessly. Are all carers supposed to be saints?

No, you do not have to be a saint. Neither are other carers. You are an ordinary person doing your best at a very difficult task. Repetitive behaviour – such as endlessly asking the same questions, shouting or misplacing things – is common among people with dementia and can be intensely irritating. It is not surprising that you sometimes lose your temper and feel that only a saint could go on.

Losing your temper probably isn't good for you and it certainly doesn't help your mother. Try to understand your mother's behaviour and see if you can stop it or reduce it (see Chapter 7 for suggestions). If you do feel you are going to lose your temper, try going into another room or into the garden. Perhaps you will be able to scream or cry there, or just take a deep breath and calm down.

You don't have to manage these problems alone. Both the

Alzheimer's Society and Alzheimer Scotland have helplines (contact details in Appendix 1). Best of all, try to get advice from your doctor or from the local community mental health nurse (see 'Services for people at home' in Chapter 9) on ways of dealing with your mother's repetitive behaviour. Also make sure you ask for regular respite breaks (see 'Respite care' in Chapter 9).

My husband keeps wandering off and being brought back by the police. I get so angry and often end up shouting at him. I know this is not good for either of us. What should I do?

It is very natural to get angry in these circumstances. Anger is a common reaction after worry. You probably get angry at your husband because you have been very worried about him, fearing that something dreadful might have happened. You just have to tell yourself that your husband can't help it. Wandering is very common in people with dementia (also see the section 'Wandering' in Chapter 6). Whenever your husband is brought back home, he is likely to be very confused and frightened. Rather than being angry with him, try very hard to reassure him and comfort him and get him back into his familiar routine.

My husband follows me from room to room and even when I go to the toilet he stands outside the door. I feel I never have any space for myself, and this makes me very tense and prone to lose my temper at him. What can I do?

Your husband is following you around because he feels insecure. He probably thinks you are not going to return and that makes him feel very unhappy.

Whenever you leave the room, it is important to try to reassure your husband that you will be coming back in a few minutes. However, to get more space and time for yourself, it would be a good idea to ask a friend or a neighbour to sit with your husband sometimes. This will probably help you to feel more relaxed and may make it easier to cope with your husband's clinging behaviour when you return.

> *I don't mind looking after my mother, who has Alzheimer's and can't manage on her own, but I feel very bitter about my brother and his wife. They won't have her to stay and never come to visit. I've given up my job, so we are on one income but my brother doesn't contribute anything financially. I think he last rang three months ago. What can I do about this?*

Alzheimer's disease doesn't just affect the person who is ill, it affects the whole family and many different relationships. Sometimes one member of the family, like you, shoulders the whole burden, while others, like your brother, keep away and pretend the problems are not their responsibility. This often leads to bitterness and family feuds.

If you can possibly manage to see your brother and talk to him, you should do so. It may be that he is finding the situation difficult, that he thinks you are much more caring than he is, or that he cannot accept your mother's illness.

If you cannot find a way for your brother to be involved, it would be better to look actively for help from elsewhere. Make sure you have all the breaks and respite care (see 'Respite care' in Chapter 9) you need. Ask your social worker to help with any benefits you can claim (also see 'State benefits' in Chapter 11). If you really look after yourself, you may feel less stressed and less bitter about your brother.

SEXUAL FEELINGS

My husband, who has Alzheimer's disease, seems to have lost all interest in having a sexual relationship with me. I miss this aspect of my life and feel very guilty about feeling this way. What can I do?

It is very natural for you to feel this way. Everyone has a life-long need to be loved and touched, and sexuality is a normal part of adult life. Gentle cuddling and holding may be mutually satisfying, and will let you know if your husband is able or inclined to engage in further intimacy. Patience may pay off. Your husband's condition may vary from time to time and there may be days when he is more sexually inclined than others.

In this situation, some people find other sexual outlets, for example masturbation or another relationship.

I have met a new friend through the carers' group I attend. We are becoming very close and I don't know what to do. My wife no longer recognises me although I care for her, but I also care for my new friend a lot. Is it wrong to start a new relationship while my wife is still alive? I think this friendship helps me care better.

This is an understandable thing to have happened. A shared experience often brings people closely together. You should talk to your new friend about her feelings as she is probably in the same situation. You need to work out how to support each other as well as your partners.

GUILT

My wife has had Alzheimer's disease for eight years and I am feeling worn out in spite of a great deal of support. I know I should consider putting her in a home but I do not know how I am going to cope with the guilt of giving up caring. Can you advise me?

You have cared for your wife already for a very long time. Also, you have loved her and know her better than anyone else does. I am sure you always felt you would be able to continue to care for her indefinitely. Unfortunately, caring for someone with Alzheimer's disease becomes a 24-hour occupation and it is not normal for anyone to continue to care on this basis without any relief. I expect you have already had help from health services and Social Services and from your local Alzheimer's Society group. However, there comes a time when short breaks of respite care just do not provide sufficient relief.

You should try to visit some homes and then introduce your wife to one of them gradually, getting her to stay there for short periods of time. Many homes are prepared to do this. In that way, the staff get to know her. If she goes there permanently, it should be possible for you to continue to care for your wife by helping at mealtimes and washing her. You can distract her and take her out and continue to contribute a great deal to her life. At the same time, you will be giving the staff of the home a great deal of support. After all, I am sure you feel that your wife would not have wanted you to risk your own health by looking after her.

Since I put my mother in a nursing home I have felt such guilt.
She was impossible to look after at home and we have two young
children. But I can't get her distress over the move out of my
mind. Have I done the wrong thing?

The decision to move someone they love into a care home is often one of the most difficult and painful decisions that carers ever have to make. You have many responsibilities, to your children and to your husband as well as to your mother. Sometimes it is not possible for people to balance their various responsibilities, and hard decisions have to be taken. Sometimes your own needs have to come first. Sometimes the needs of the person you love are so complex that you cannot provide good care for them at home.

Face up to the decision and think about the advantages for you, your mother and your family. Try to concentrate on the positive care your mother is getting at the care home. Visit her as much as possible and encourage other members of the family and her friends to visit her too. Make sure she knows you haven't forgotten her and that you and the family still love her. Take your children with you if you can.

9 | Getting help

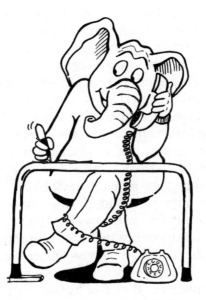

Getting the help that is needed when you or someone you care for has Alzheimer's disease or another dementia is not always easy. There is a wide range of information and advice, services and support, but finding your way through to the different organisations and agencies that provide it can be difficult. The three key contacts are the GP of the person with dementia, the local Social Services and the Alzheimer's Society. There are also many other local organisations and groups. This chapter answers common questions about types of help and how to get it.

SOURCES OF HELP AND INFORMATION

Where can I turn to for help and information?

Many people and organisations, both professional and voluntary, can help make your life easier. Don't be afraid to ask. You will find a list of useful addresses and telephone numbers in Appendix 1, including those of the organisations mentioned below.

The Alzheimer's Society is there to help everyone affected by dementia of whatever type. This is true of Alzheimer associations world-wide. Your local branch will know about local services. It will also have as members many carers and some people with dementia, who will understand your worries and problems and be able to help you. If you join the Society, you will receive a useful monthly newsletter full of news and practical advice.

Carers UK is a support organisation for carers of all kinds. The Princess Royal Trust for Carers has many Carers' Centres which give information. Age Concern will also help you. Expert advice on benefits can be obtained from Citizens Advice. Everyone who needs care is entitled to a multi-disciplinary assessment of their needs, which may be initiated by the GP or by your local authority's Social Services. The person caring for you is also entitled to have his or her needs assessed separately (for more information about needs assessments, see the section 'Community care' later in this chapter).

Are there training courses for people caring for someone with dementia?

There are many opportunities for family carers to learn about dementia and how to care for someone who has it. Branches of the Alzheimer's Society (contact details in Appendix 1) and local carers' groups often have speakers and may run practical sessions on topics such as difficult behaviour, safety aspects or lifting people. In some areas, more formal courses are run by Social Services to help carers with their task. Alzheimer Scotland and the Alzheimer's Society in Northern Ireland have specific training courses for carers. Video training materials are also available from a number of different sources. There are also many conferences for carers, organised at regional and national level. You can find out about these from the Alzheimer's Society Newsletter or from Alzheimer Scotland (contact details in Appendix 1).

I have recently been told I am in the early stages of dementia. Is there a group I can go to, or somewhere to meet other people like myself?

There are support groups for people with dementia. These groups meet regularly and you can talk about your feelings, exchange tips about managing your memory loss and perhaps go on outings and trips together. Contact the Alzheimer's Society or Alzheimer Scotland for support, and to find out whether there is a group near you.

SPIRITUAL NEEDS

My husband and I have always gone to our church on Sundays. Although he doesn't understand much now, he still seems to enjoy the services and to benefit from them. I worry about other people, though, as he makes disturbing noises. Can you advise me?

If you have a religious faith, you will believe that a person with dementia retains their spiritual dimension intact despite the disease. It is right, therefore, to try to meet those spiritual needs. The ritual of familiar religious services can be very helpful and calming for a person with dementia, and people should be given the opportunity to attend their place of worship for as long as they are able. The minister and other worshippers will probably be very tolerant and helpful if you explain the situation to them.

When someone with dementia is no longer able to go out, a minister will visit them at home and say prayers or give the sacraments as appropriate.

The Christian Council on Ageing is concerned with the spiritual needs of people with dementia. It publishes some useful guides. Jewish Care may also be able to help. (See Appendix 1.)

How can we try to meet the spiritual needs of people with dementia?

People get a sense of happiness and well-being from many artistic and religious experiences. It may be through practice of faith, but also through music and the arts, gardening and the enjoyment of nature. They can all speak to the person within. People at all stages of dementia have the capacity to enjoy these things.

COMMUNITY CARE

How do I get help with caring at home?

'Community care' is a general term for services provided to help people with illness or disability to continue to live in their own homes and to encourage independence. The policy of community care also encourages the local provision of sheltered housing and of residential and nursing homes (care homes) within the general community.

Legislation confirms Social Services departments' responsibility to assess people's needs (by a procedure known as a *needs assessment*, discussed below) and to provide or purchase a range of services to meet those needs. The aim is that services will be provided to keep people in their own homes for as long as possible.

There are a number of different services designed to support people in their own homes. However, the range and level of services vary a great deal from area to area. You may have to be determined to get enough care for someone to be supported at home. Local authorities are not legally obliged to provide community care for individuals if this would cost more than moving them to a residential or nursing home, although they sometimes will.

To obtain services provided by the NHS – such as nursing help or physiotherapy – you should ask the GP or hospital specialist of the person who is ill. To obtain other services – such as home care assistants ('home helps') or meals on wheels – first ask your Social Services department for a needs assessment. Then ask Social Services what they should and can provide to meet those needs. You can find out whom to speak to by ringing the local Council offices. (See the section 'Services for people at home' later in this chapter for information about the different types of services that might be available.)

I've been told I'm to have a 'needs assessment' for community care. What is this?

A needs assessment is organised by Social Services when they think that someone may need community care. The assessment will usually be carried out by a social worker or an occupational therapist. They will talk to you and take account of the views of your GP and community mental health nurse if you have one. Your carer, or a close relative, should also be able to be involved and to contribute. (Carers can also request a needs assessment; see later in this section.)

The needs assessment will include reports from the various professionals who have been involved. It may also include a questionnaire. You need to be sure that the questionnaire is properly filled in. You should ask for assurance that the assessment system being used is appropriate for people with dementia. If in doubt, contact the Alzheimer's Society.

After a needs assessment has been carried out, your 'key worker' – who may be a social worker or a nurse or a care manager – should discuss with you what services are available in your area to meet your needs. The care manager (see the next answer) will draw up and monitor a care plan for you.

What is a care manager?

A care manager, usually a social worker, is a person who draws up and manages a care plan for someone who has had a needs assessment (see the previous answer). The care plan sets out the types of community care that should be available to meet the needs of the person who has been assessed.

The care manager is an important person for you to work with. A good care manager will be very supportive and a useful source of information and advice. The care manager should provide a copy of the needs assessment and also of the care plan, and be prepared to discuss them with you. He or she should monitor the care plan and make appropriate changes to it to meet changing needs. If you do not see your care manager on a regular basis, you should contact him or her whenever your needs change.

What can I do if I don't agree with the needs assessment or with the amount of help offered for my father, who has dementia?

If you do not agree with the needs assessment or with the care plan for your father, you should discuss the problem with his care manager. If you cannot reach an agreement with your father's care manager, you should follow the complaints procedure which will be published by your Social Services department or the Patient Advice and Liaison Service (PALS) of your NHS Trust.

My mother has Alzheimer's disease but her GP isn't very helpful. The GP says my mother should go into a nursing home. My father wants my mother to stay at home with him. If this is to happen he needs a lot more help. What can I do?

The first step is for you to think very carefully about whether your father is likely to be able to cope with looking after your mother, and for how long. You also need to think about how much extra help might be needed to enable him to do this.

The GP's opinion may be valuable, but it is really for your family to decide together with Social Services what is best. You should ask Social Services for an assessment (or reassessment) of your mother's needs or a separate assessment for your father (see the section 'Services for people at home' later in this chapter).

If a decision is made to keep your mother at home, and her GP is still unhappy about this, you may want to discuss it with the GP so that he or she understands your position better. You may like to take someone from the Alzheimer's Society with you to help the discussion. Even so, you should probably start thinking ahead to a time when your mother may be better off in a nursing home (see Chapter 10).

A few years ago I had a slight stroke. It has left me very weak on one side and a bit wobbly. Now my wife is getting confused. The doctor says it's Alzheimer's disease. We want to go on caring for each other but I'm scared of the future. How can I care for her if I'm disabled myself?

If you have not already done so, ask Social Services to conduct a needs assessment under the Community Care Act. They should assess your and your wife's needs both as people with care needs and as carers (see the section 'Services for people at home' later in this chapter). Make sure also that you are getting all the state benefits, such as Attendance Allowance, that you are entitled to (see the section 'State benefits' in Chapter 11).

The fact that your stroke has left you with strength and mobility problems will make some things more difficult for you, and where you live will make a lot of difference. You might want to consider moving into sheltered housing (see the next answer).

Try to make a realistic assessment of what you can and can't do and remember that your wife will need a lot more care later in her illness. With extra help, you and she may be able to continue caring for each other for a time. However, this may not be possible indefinitely, because her needs and perhaps also yours may become too great. Taking time now to make practical plans for the future, such as investigating a possible move either into sheltered housing or into a care home (see Chapter 10), is itself an important aspect of caring for someone.

I want to carry on looking after my husband, who has dementia, but my arthritis is making me less mobile. Might a move to sheltered housing be the answer?

This type of accommodation is designed specially for people with mobility and care needs. Residents continue to live as independently as possible, in self-contained flats or in a complex of houses. The units may have fittings, such as easy-to-use taps and safety rails, to help people with mobility problems. They also have alarms for calling a warden in case of emergency. There might also be Social Services help with shopping, cooking and so on. There are some places now that are able to give more help as people's needs increase.

My neighbour, who lives alone, is getting very confused. I try to keep an eye on him but I'm worried about his safety. What if he leaves the gas on? He doesn't seem to have any relatives. Whom should I contact?

If Social Services are already helping your neighbour, for example if he has a home care assistant ('home help') or receives meals on wheels, you should share your safety fears with them.

You can contact Social Services, even if they are not involved, if you are worried about your neighbour's safety.

On the specific question of gas safety, gas suppliers keep a register of customers who need special attention and special services. There are now various gadgets that help with home safety. If it is really not possible to ensure the safety of your neighbour, it may be necessary for Social Services to disconnect the cooker and to arrange for a home care assistant or meals on wheels to provide food.

My father, who has dementia, can no longer cope on his own but he refuses to move out of his flat. A social worker told me that my father may be 'Sectioned'. What does this mean?

Sometimes people with dementia may behave in ways that put their own safety or the safety of others at risk. For example, your father may be leaving the gas on or wandering the streets in the middle of the night. Such behaviour is especially dangerous when someone is living alone.

If the social workers and doctors involved consider that it is no longer safe for someone with dementia to live alone, they will first try to persuade them to go into some form of care, where they would be safer. However, some people with dementia don't realise they have a problem and are reluctant to leave their home. Striking a balance between their safety, the safety of others and their freedom is not easy.

As a last resort, the social workers and doctors involved with someone they consider to be at risk can force that person to go into a hospital or a care home. This is the process commonly known as 'sectioning', because it uses powers under a section of the Mental Health Act 1983 for England and Wales. The terms of the section allow a person at risk to be taken to a place of safety without their consent. This is an uncommon step, which is not taken lightly. It may, however, be necessary in extreme situations.

SERVICES FOR PEOPLE AT HOME

I have been diagnosed with Alzheimer's disease. My partner would like to try to care for me at home. What sort of services might be available? Will we have to pay?

It is generally thought that people should be helped to remain in their own homes for as long as possible if that is their wish. However, some local health authorities and Social Services offer more community care than others. A person who would be able to continue to live at home with the amount of support provided in some places might not be able to do so elsewhere. The extent to which people are expected to pay for community care services also varies from place to place. It is common for charges to be made for services, depending on the income and savings. There may be waiting lists. Services sometimes provided at home include:

- home care assistants ('home helps') (see also the next answer);
- meals on wheels;
- continence advice and special laundry services;
- advice on aids to increase safety in the home (see the section 'Dangers at home' in Chapter 6);
- equipment (e.g. a bath seat);
- home care;
- different types of nursing care;
- physiotherapy to help with mobility;
- chiropody;
- speech and language therapy;
- day centres;
- respite care.

Some services have to be provided wherever you live if the needs assessment recognises you need them. These include home care assistants, day centres, meals on wheels and aids in the home.

Social Services are going to provide a 'home help' because my
husband has Alzheimer's disease. What sort of jobs will she do?

The type of work done by 'home helps' – home care assistants –
varies, according to need and also according to local Social
Services provisions. Your husband's care manager (explained in the
previous section) will be able to tell you exactly what to expect. Jobs
often done by 'home helps' include light housework and shopping.
Some of them also help with aspects of personal care, such as
getting up in the morning, getting ready for bed in the evening, and
at mealtimes.

My wife has had Alzheimer's disease for some time now and I
am beginning to realise that I may soon need some more help
with looking after her. What sort of nursing care might be
available on the NHS, and who should I speak to?

Your wife's GP or hospital specialist will be able to tell you about
the nursing services that might be available to help you look
after your wife. The way that community nursing services are
organised – and also their availability – varies from one area to
another. There may be a long waiting list.

When someone with Alzheimer's disease is living at home, various community-based nurses may become involved. The most
important of these tends to be the community mental health nurse
(formerly called community psychiatric nurse, or CPN). These
nurses work as part of a team that includes psychiatrists specialising
in the care of older people. They are sometimes involved in needs
assessments (discussed in the earlier section, 'Community care'), and
they may also make visits to monitor patients who have dementia
and to give advice and help to carers. Community mental health
nurses also liaise with other specialists about arranging respite care
(discussed later in this chapter), continence advice, district nursing,
support for carers, and so on.

The other community-based nurse who often becomes involved

when someone has Alzheimer's disease is the district nurse. These nurses have had special training in supporting people at home. They provide practical nursing care, such as changing wound dressings, supervising medication and giving injections. The District Nursing Service will also provide advice on equipment and aids, particularly continence aids. Community matrons have a specific role in supporting people with long-term conditions in their own homes.

Are there any specialist Alzheimer's nurses who might be able to help me?

In some places there are specialist nurses called Admiral nurses, who are trained to look after the carers of people with Alzheimer's disease. If you want to know if there is an Admiral nurse in your area, contact For Dementia (address in Appendix 1).

DAY CARE

I am unhappy to leave my mother alone all day when I am out at work. She has Alzheimer's disease. Could she go to a day centre?

Many areas have day centres that provide day care for people with Alzheimer's disease and other dementias. These are mainly run by voluntary organisations, sometimes by Social Services or less commonly by the local Primary Care Trust (when they may be known as a day hospital). You can can find out about local day care by speaking to Social Services or contacting local voluntary organisations, such as the Alzheimer's Society or Age Concern. Sometimes, day care is provided by nursing homes.

Day centres can allow carers to continue to work or to have some time to themselves, while providing the person who has Alzheimer's disease with appropriate care away from home. However, the quality of day care varies. Before your mother starts attending a centre, make sure there are suitable rooms, that the staff are well trained, that there are interesting and relevant activities (see the section 'Activities' in Chapter 5) during the day and that the food is varied and nice to eat. You should be given proper information by the day care manager about what to expect from the centre and how to complain if you are not satisfied. Your mother should have a personal care plan prepared by the centre, which takes into account her interests and needs.

Transport should be available to and from day care. Try to avoid long travelling times – more than an hour can leave people more confused and tired. A charge may be made for day care and also for transport and food, depending on your mother's income and savings.

My sister, who has dementia, refuses to go to the day centre.
I am over 80 myself and can't cope with her on my own all day.
Might it be possible for someone to come in and help care for her
at home?

Before making other arrangements for your sister, it would be worth seeing if you can find out why she doesn't like the day centre. It is possible, for example, that a change of transport, or your accompanying her on a few occasions, or a change in her activities at the centre could make it more acceptable.

If the day centre really is not possible, home care is an alternative in many areas. Home care is sometimes called a sitting service, but good home care is a lot more than just sitting. A care worker will come into your home and look after the person with dementia while you have a rest, do the shopping, visit friends or just do what you want to do.

Home care is usually arranged for part of a day and paid for on an hourly basis. It is provided by Social Services, by voluntary organisations such as Crossroads Care Attendants Schemes (contact details in Appendix 1), and by private agencies. Make sure that any agency you use has well-trained staff who know about dementia. Members of the United Kingdom Home Care Association (contact details in Appendix 1) have a code of practice.

Some home care agency staff also take people with dementia out – for a walk to the park, on visits or shopping. Voluntary organisations often arrange trips out for groups.

RESPITE CARE

What is respite care and how do I get it?

Respite care means having someone look after the person you are caring for to give you both a break. A break from caring is very important for you and for the person you are caring for. You can find out about respite care provision in your area by asking Social Services or the GP or hospital consultant of the person you care for.

Respite care can take a number of forms. Usually, a person with dementia will go into a hospital or care home for a week or two. In some areas, 'home respite' is available. This means that people move into your home for a time to look after the person with dementia so that you can have a break. Private nursing homes also sometimes offer respite care. This is not a bad way of trying out a nursing home that may be needed in the future.

As a carer you have a right to a carer's assessment (see the section 'Community care', earlier). Ask Social Services for an assessment of your needs and request that a break from caring is arranged for you. You will probably have to pay something towards the cost of Social Services respite, but it is worth arguing about payment, as they do have discretion over this.

People with dementia may find it difficult to settle into respite care. It is a matter of trial and error, and you will need to be sure that the needs of the person you care for are really understood. It may be difficult, but remember that respite is in your and their long-term interests.

I am 70 and looking after my wife who has Alzheimer's. Recently I had flu and couldn't cope. Luckily my sister came round and helped look after us both. But what could I do if my sister weren't there?

You cannot care for someone properly if you are ill yourself. If necessary, your wife could go into emergency respite care. Your Care Manager, social worker or Community Matron would be able to organise this. Most Social Service departments have special facilities for just such emergencies, and your wife could be admitted to a respite bed at very short notice.

10 | Residential and nursing homes

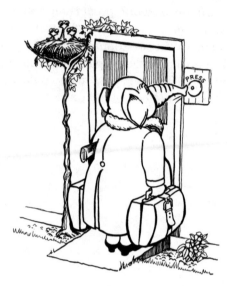

Most people with dementia will eventually need to go into a care home. They may need very intensive care, and the demands of looking after someone with dementia day in day out over a long period of time usually become too great for most family carers, however much they may love the person who is ill. This chapter describes the two types of care home: residential (sometimes called just 'care home') and nursing (sometimes called 'care home (nursing)'). It also gives useful advice on what to look for when choosing a home and on how to make the move into the home as easy as possible.

IS A HOME NECESSARY?

My husband who has dementia was taken into hospital because he has become incontinent and I cannot go on looking after him at home. The hospital now says he has to be put in a nursing home. I think he would be better cared for in hospital. Can they ask him to leave against my will?

Very few people with dementia are now cared for in hospital on a long-term basis. People are sometimes admitted to hospital for assessment or because of a problem such as a fall. NHS continuing care is only provided if they need frequent supervision by a hospital consultant or constant specialist nursing. NHS continuing care is now normally provided in nursing homes.

If a person is considered not to require NHS continuing care, they have no right to stay in hospital. They do, however, have a right to refuse to be sent to a residential or nursing home for which they will have to pay.

Before the hospital can move your husband, it must arrange a multi-disciplinary assessment of his needs. The assessment should involve staff from the hospital, your husband's GP and also Social Services (assessment is described on page 140). Your husband's view, if possible, and also your view must be taken into account.

If your husband comes back to your home, Social Services must arrange care. (Community care is discussed in Chapter 9.)

The hospital consultant has the final decision as to whether your husband should stay in hospital. There are locally agreed criteria based on national guidelines for NHS continuing care. If you are unhappy about the decision, you can appeal, but only if the guidelines have not been followed correctly; you cannot appeal against the guidelines themselves. The person who advises you about the decision should be able to tell you how to appeal. The Alzheimer's Society Helpline (see Appendix 1) can also provide information about NHS continuing care.

My aunt, when she was dying of cancer, was cared for very well in a hospice. Can hospices look after people with dementia?

The hospice movement was started to provide special care for people who are dying. Over the years it has developed great expertise in controlling pain and in helping people to take control of their own deaths.

Hospices are not really suitable for people with dementia because much of their work and skills are directed towards helping patients to make choices for themselves and to face up to their own terminal illness. At the end of their lives, people with dementia are not able to act in this way.

It is true, however, that care homes that care for people with dementia at the end of their lives have things to learn from the hospice movement. Respect, dignity, choice and acceptance of death are all of value to people with dementia and those who love them. The best doctors, nurses and care workers know this and, wherever they are working, try hard to provide the right kind of care for people with dementia who are dying.

The staff in a good care home will be able to talk to you about how they deal with dying and the special care they give people at the end of their lives.

I did not wish to put my husband with Alzheimer's disease into a home so early on. It was hell with him at home as I still have children living here, but then it is hell seeing him in the nursing home. There is no answer . . . or is there?

It is common to feel guilty when someone close to you has to go into a care home. You probably feel guilty because in a residential or nursing home the care is not going to be so personal and you may feel you have let your husband down. This may be made worse by reproach from your husband, who probably does not understand that you simply could not manage him in your own home.

The most important way to respond to feelings of guilt is to recognise the way you feel so that you are able to make clear-headed decisions about the future and what is right for the whole family. You should also realise that nothing you did or didn't do could have prevented the disease. You cannot influence the timing or the eventual outcome of Alzheimer's disease. All you can do is to ensure that your husband is comfortable, safe and reasonably content.

Try to get along to a carers' support group. You may be surprised how many people feel as you do.

INFORMATION SOURCES

I think the time has come to look for a nursing home for my mother, who has dementia. How do I find out about nursing homes in the area where she lives?

Many GP practices have lists of local care homes and some information about them. Your Social Services should also have such a list. However, these lists will often do no more than give the names and addresses of homes, so you will need to find out for yourself which homes look after people with dementia.

Another option is to contact the Elderly Accommodation Council (contact details in Appendix 1). This organisation will send you a questionnaire to fill in and, for a small fee, will send a list of homes that might meet your requirements. The Alzheimer's Society Helpline can also help with information on homes for people with dementia.

There are also various commercially produced directories, some with the support of Social Services departments. These directories contain useful information but it is important to remember that they are compiled on the basis of information from the home owners and are funded by advertising. They sometimes give the impression that they can recommend homes but you must make your own best judgement.

None of these lists or directories inspects or recommends homes. It is important to remember that no list can be completely accurate or up to date. You will still have to find out for yourselves what is suitable and also what your mother can afford or Social Services will pay for. Your mother's nursing care, if she needs it, will be assessed and paid for (see the last answer in the next section, 'Types of homes'). It can be very time-consuming visiting homes and trying to choose a good one, but it is usually worth the effort. Also try asking people you know if they can make any recommendations. Early planning is important because good homes are often full and there may be waiting lists.

The Commission for Social Care Inspection (contact details in Appendix 1), which is the official body that regulates care homes, publishes its reports on its website. You can find out about care homes in your area and also what the inspectors thought of them.

TYPES OF HOMES

What is the difference between residential homes and nursing homes, and are only nursing homes suitable for people with dementia?

The main difference between residential and nursing homes (also called 'care home' and 'care home (nursing)') is that residential homes do not have to have nurses on the staff, whereas nursing homes must employ qualified nurses and must be able to provide 24-hour nursing care.

Some residential homes, which have real commitment and well-trained staff, can care very well for people with dementia. (People with dementia make up some two-thirds of all the people currently in these two types of care home.) In general, residential homes look after people who are more active and alert. Residential homes will help them with washing, dressing and toileting and of course provide meals and activities. Sometimes, a residential home will allow a person to stay on there even though they have developed dementia or become more frail. There will, however, be less nursing care than would be available in a nursing home.

People with dementia who also have physical and/or challenging behaviour will probably need the level of care provided by a nursing home. It may also be better for people without these added problems to go straight into a nursing home, to avoid the disruption of having to move them again at a later date. Many people in nursing homes will have some dementia. Some nursing homes specialise in caring for people with dementia. People who are very difficult to care for will need to go into a specialist nursing home or to be looked after in an NHS hospital.

The real difference is in the way care is paid for. Care provided by a registered nurse is free to the resident, so nursing homes are paid that cost by the NHS.

Who usually provides residential homes and nursing homes, and how are they regulated?

Sometimes a local authority has its own residential homes (sometimes called 'part III homes') but these are becoming less and less common. Other residential homes are provided by private organisations or individuals or on a not-for-profit basis by registered charities or religious organisations.

Most nursing homes are privately owned by individuals or, increasingly, by big companies. Some are run by charities. Nursing homes are usually more expensive than residential homes because of the nursing care that they provide.

Some homes have dual registration as providing both residential and nursing care. It has been suggested that the distinction between residential and nursing home care is a false one, particularly as most older people need more care as time goes on and it is not sensible for them to have to move.

All care homes are regulated and inspected by the Commission for Social Care Inspection.

I've been told my father has to have an assessment before he goes into a nursing home. What does this mean, and will I have a say in where he goes?

All people in need of health and social care should now go through a single assessment process. The aim is to ensure that all their needs are identified so that arrangements can be made to care for them. The assessment has two stages: a multi-disciplinary assessment of needs and, if the person needs nursing home care, an assessment of registered nursing input.

The *multi-disciplinary assessment* should look at your father's physical health, his mental health, especially his dementia, and his social needs. The aim should be to keep him independent as long as possible.

If he is assessed as needing to be in a nursing home, there will be a second *assessment of registered nursing input* to his care. This assessment is to decide how much financial contribution the NHS will make to his nursing home.

If your father is paying the full cost of his care, it is his and your choice where he goes. If Social Services are paying, they should consult you but the choice of home will depend on what is available and how much they will pay.

CHOOSING A HOME

My father lives alone and has Alzheimer's disease. Even with a 'home help' he cannot manage on his own any more. What should I look for when choosing a home for him?

First you need to know that the home will take people with dementia and knows how to look after them. Your father's care manager, social worker, GP, consultant or community mental health nurse may be able to make suggestions, as will the nearest branch of the Alzheimer's Society. When you have some names and addresses, you can write or telephone to find out about the level of care provided, the fees and if a place is available. Many homes will send a brochure but you should check the facts for yourself.

If you can, make appointments to visit several homes, and at different times of the day, before choosing one. Even two homes offering exactly the same level of care can have a quite different atmosphere. When you have a short-list of homes, take your father to visit them if you possibly can. After all, it will be his home and he has a right to choose as far as he is able.

Choosing a suitable home is a matter of observing carefully and asking lots of questions. Speak to the person in charge and also to members of staff. Try to assess how knowledgeable they are, especially about the needs of people with dementia. Do staff acknowledge residents courteously and by name? Do residents look relaxed and engaged with life? Also, if possible, try to speak to other residents and their families to find out what they think about the care offered.

Some questions to consider when choosing are:

- Where is the home situated? Will it be easy for friends and family to visit?

- Are there places to get out to? Are outings arranged?

- Is there a safe garden to walk in?

- Is the home friendly, welcoming and homely?

- Is it well furnished?

- Are there enough rooms for residents to sit in?

- Is it clean and sweet smelling? There should be no smell of urine.

- What is the home's practice about smoking? (The law states that residents may smoke in their own room but staff and visitors are not allowed to smoke on the premises.)

- Are there activities going on? How are chairs arranged?

- Is the television just left on all day?

- Is there access for wheelchairs or walking frames? Are there suitably adapted toilets and baths?

- Can your father have a single room if that is what he would prefer?

- Can he bring his own furniture and other possessions?

- Can residents use their own rooms to be private and do staff respect their need for privacy?

- Will he have his own toilet? Are there enough toilets and bathrooms for all the residents?

- Do the staff treat people with tact and respect when helping them with bathing or using the toilet?

- What is the food like? Is the food at the home appealing and nutritious? Are choices offered at meal-times? Does the home cater for special diets? (What we eat and when we eat it is an important factor in quality of life.)

- Will your father be able to eat in his room if he wishes?

- Will he be able to eat at a different time, or have a snack, just like in his own home?

- What are the arrangements for medical care?

- Are dental treatment and chiropody available?

- Is there evidence that every person is cared for as an individual?

If you feel that you need more detailed advice on choosing a home, further information is available from Age Concern, the Alzheimer's Society, Counsel and Care, and the Relatives and Residents Association (contact details in Appendix 1).

Do the staff running a care home have to be properly qualified? How can I find out if they are trained to do the job?

All care homes (residential and nursing) have to be registered with the Commission for Social Care Inspection. All nursing homes are required to have a qualified nurse on duty at all times, but apart from this there are no requirements for care homes to be owned by, or to employ, qualified staff.

When choosing a care home, you should ask the owner or manager what qualifications they or other senior staff have and what arrangements are made for staff training. You should also make a point of asking if they have particular knowledge of looking after people with dementia. Apart from general nursing qualifications, psychiatric nursing or social work qualifications are relevant. It would also be useful to know if there is an occupational therapist either on the staff or coming into the home regularly. The home should have its own training programme for care staff; for instance, staff might follow the Alzheimer's Society care learning programme and be Alzheimer's Society certified care workers.

You can tell a lot from the way staff in a home behave. Are they sensitive, tolerant and caring as well as efficient, hardworking and capable? Good care is a matter of natural ability as well as training.

MAKING THE MOVE

It must be very upsetting to have to move from your own home into a care home. What is the best way of preparing for this and arranging it so that my mother is distressed as little as possible?

Good planning and preparation are the best way of minimising distress for people when they move. Often, people go into a care home when there is a crisis and that makes things more difficult for everyone. It is important to face up in advance to the likelihood that residential or nursing home care will be needed eventually.

Find out about suitable homes in your area and visit them all. Take your mother with you if she is able. It will be her home, so as far as possible she should choose. It might help if your mother could go to a home for day care, perhaps one day a week or more for a while, so that she can see if she likes it and get used to the people.

Another possibility might be for your mother to take advantage of a home's provision of respite breaks and stay there for a week occasionally. This can have benefits for all concerned. Your mother will become familiar with the people and the place, you will know whether or not she likes it, and the staff will find out about her needs. A series of short stays of this kind, preparing for a permanent move, will also help you to discover if the care in the home is good. It's not always possible to do as much preparation as this but do try to make sure that your mother visits different homes and has some choice.

It will probably be helpful if you can visit your mother often when she first moves into the home, and do try to make sure she knows when you will be returning. Also make sure that she has some of her own furniture and some familiar objects, such as ornaments and photographs, with her.

This can be a very distressing and difficult time for everyone, but handled well it will bring security for your mother and a sense of release for you as a carer.

PRIVACY OR COMPANY?

It seems to me to be quite wrong that my sister, who has Alzheimer's disease, is put in a room by herself in the nursing home. She can hardly communicate and she needs company. I think she would benefit from sharing a room with other people.

Everyone is different, but it is thought to be better for most people in nursing homes to have their own bedrooms rather than needing to share with a stranger. Having your own bedroom means that privacy and dignity can be maintained at all times, particularly when intimate care and personal tasks are involved. All homes are now required to provide single rooms for residents.

Having your own bedroom shouldn't mean you are alone. People should be out of bed and staff should be talking to them and involving them as far as is possible in the life of the care home. If your sister is just being left alone in bed for long periods, the home is not caring for her very well. You should speak to the home manager if you think this is the case.

Obviously there are a few people who like company so much that they enjoy being with others all the time. Shared rooms are sometimes provided in homes, usually at a lower cost, and if you are sure that this is what your sister would like, even though she is now ill, you may be able to arrange it for her.

POSSIBLE ILL-TREATMENT

My father is in a home. He has severe dementia and needs a great deal of care. The last couple of times I have visited him I have noticed bruises on his arms. The staff all seem very nice but I'm worried that someone may be being rough with him. What should I do?

You are right to be concerned but people with dementia may have bruises for a number of quite innocent reasons. Older people have fragile skin that tends to bruise with little pressure. Your father may be unsteady on his feet and bump into things or fall. It is possible that he may have become involved in a disagreement with another resident. However, the fact remains that older people are sometimes at risk from ill-treatment or neglect by a care worker.

If you suspect that your father is being ill treated in the home, there are several things you should do. First, try to see as much as possible of your father's skin (you could say you want to bath him) and look for bruises elsewhere. Also, glance at other residents to see whether anyone else has bruises. If you are still concerned, write down the dates of your visits and the location of your father's bruises. You should then take this information with you and ask the home manager for an explanation. If the home manager fails to provide you with a satisfactory reply, speak to your father's care manager or social worker or to the Commission for Social Care Inspection (contact details in Appendix 1).

In cases of suspected ill-treatment it can be tempting to say nothing, for fear of causing more problems. However, if any ill-treatment is taking place it must be investigated. Ultimately, you may feel that your father is best moved to another home, where the staff are better trained and better supervised.

VISITING

My wife is now in a nursing home because of her Alzheimer's disease. I try to visit her every day but I am finding this quite exhausting. Do you think it matters if I do not visit her quite so often?

You have probably found it very difficult to accept that you cannot look after your wife any more at home. You may feel that you have let her down and you are perhaps blaming yourself for not being able to manage. The care your wife is receiving in the nursing home will not, of course, be as personal and may not be as good as the care you were giving her at home. Many carers want to go on helping as much as they possibly can. It will probably take you a while to come to terms with the fact that your wife is quite well cared for in the home and does seem fairly content and comfortable when you visit.

Your wife is very unlikely to remember exactly when you last visited. You and your wife will enjoy your visits much more if you are less tired and more cheerful, and it sounds as if you could do with taking a break and putting trust in the people who are now looking after your wife. You will probably find it helpful to talk with one or two of the staff about how you are feeling and tell them that you are going to visit less often. Let the staff know that you support their caring role, and they will support you.

11 | Legal and financial advice

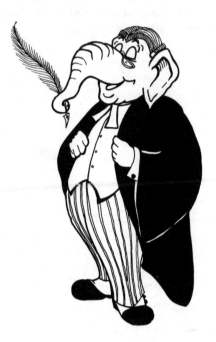

Nearly all people with Alzheimer's disease and other dementias will become unable to manage their financial affairs, and many of the people caring for them will become involved in financial or legal problems of some kind. Most of the real difficulties can be avoided or reduced by early planning. Many financial benefits are available from the state for people with dementia and their carers. However, the rules relating to them are complicated and it is important to seek individual advice. Also note that benefits and amounts often change, so the information given here is only a general guide. Your local Citizens Advice (CAB; formerly Citizens Advice Bureau) will be a very useful source of help on benefits and financial planning.

Remember, too, that if you are managing someone else's finances you should always try to involve them as much as possible. People with dementia can still make choices even if they are no longer sure of the value of things, and it is right that they should understand as much as possible of what is being decided for them.

Solicitors can be expensive and are not always necessary but a solicitor who is experienced and knowledgeable in advising older people can be very helpful and may save you money over all. The Alzheimer's Society has specialist legal and financial advisers and can put you in touch with solicitors who have received specialist training.

GETTING ADVICE

Where can I get good advice on legal and financial matters?

L egal and financial problems can be complicated and it is always wise to seek independent advice.

Your local Citizens Advice (CAB) is often the best starting point. Advice is free and confidential and the CAB staff will help to sort out your problems and give you clear information. Some CABs have specialist legal and financial advisers. The address of your local CAB should be in the telephone book. If you need specifically legal advice, Law Centres give free advice on problems such as welfare rights, state benefits, housing and employment. To find out if there is a Law Centre near you, ask at your local library or consult the phone book or internet (contact details in Appendix 1).

If you are arranging a will (see below) or a Lasting Power of Attorney (see the next section), you may wish to contact a solicitor. It may be helpful to ask for a recommendation from friends or relatives locally. The Alzheimer's Society (contact details in Appendix 1) has a list of solicitors who have specialist knowledge of the legal problems of people with dementia and their carers. If you are going to a solicitor for the first time, do not be afraid to ask for a clear written estimate of costs and an explanation of the work they will do on your behalf.

Information on state benefits can be obtained from your local Social Services department. There is also the Benefits Enquiry Line (contact details in Appendix 1). This is a free national telephone advice and information service for people with disabilities and their carers. It provides general advice on benefits but will not answer questions on your specific situation.

Advice on benefits is also available from Age Concern, the Alzheimer's Society and Alzheimer Scotland.

LEGAL SAFEGUARDS

I have recently been diagnosed with Alzheimer's disease and I want to make a will. Are there any special things I should think about?

It is very important to make a will. It is usually easy and not expensive. Making a will makes sure that your estate (your possessions) goes to those you want it to and makes it much easier to settle your affairs after you die.

If your estate is only small and your plans are simple, a postal will-making service may be adequate. However, for most people, it is best to take legal advice when making a will. Always ask in advance for an estimate of the cost of making a will. Legal advice can be obtained from a Law Centre or from a solicitor. The Alzheimer's Society has a list of solicitors who have a special interest in and knowledge of legal matters affecting people with dementia.

When planning your will, you will need to consider your personal circumstances and your relatives and friends. If you own your own house and share it with someone who is caring for you, you may want to make arrangements to protect their interest in it. You may also want to plan for nursing home fees in the future. It is not easy to think about the difficulties ahead, but if you can manage to do this and take good advice you will help not only yourself but also those you love.

A solicitor may offer to draw up a Lasting Power of Attorney (see the next answer) at the same time as making a will and have an all-inclusive price. You may think this is a good idea.

What is a Lasting Power of Attorney?

A Lasting Power of Attorney (LPA) is a legal document in which one person gives another or others the power to handle his or her personal affairs. This can only be set up when the person giving it is mentally capable of understanding what he or she is doing. For this reason, it is important for anyone who has been given a diagnosis of dementia to consider having a Lasting Power of Attorney drawn up as soon as possible. A doctor's advice may be sought if there is any doubt about a person's mental capacity. However, 'mental capacity' has a legal, not a medical, definition.

A Lasting Power of Attorney is a new legal arrangement established by the Mental Capacity Act 2005 which came into effect in October 2007. It replaces the Enduring Power of Attorney. (In Scotland a similar measure is called a Continuing Power of Attorney.) A Lasting Power of Attorney will give the recipient (the attorney) considerable power over the person's (the donor's) living arrangements, health care and finances, so it is important to choose someone the donor trusts and who is capable of making judgements in his or her best interests. People usually choose their spouse or partner or one or more of their children.

To make a Lasting Power of Attorney you need a special form, which you can get from a law stationer or solicitor, or free from the new Public Guardianship Office (contact details in Appendix 1). The form allows the donor to specify the powers that the attorney will have such as consenting to treatment on your behalf or deciding where you should live. It names the person appointed as attorney and must be signed by the attorney, the donor and at least one witness who is not a relative of the donor. It is important to use the right form and to complete it properly, otherwise the Power of Attorney will be invalid. A Lasting Power of Attorney should not be confused with an Enduring Power of Attorney, which covers only financial matters or with an ordinary Power of Attorney, which ceases to be valid when a person becomes mentally incapacitated.

When the attorney believes that the donor has become mentally incapable, he or she must notify the donor and certain close relatives of his or her intention to register the Lasting Power of Attorney. An application to register must be made to the Public Guardianship Office. The registration will take several weeks because the Office must hold the papers for 35 days to allow time for objections to be made. Registration will cost several hundred pounds; less if you do it yourself, more if you use a solicitor.

If all is in order, notice of approval is sent and the attorney is then able to act in accordance with the terms laid down by the donor.

My father has had dementia for two years. Is it still possible for him to make a will or sign a Lasting Power of Attorney?

It may still be possible, depending on your father's mental capabilities. If you are worried about your father's competence, to avoid problems in future it may be wise to consult a doctor or solicitor to ensure that your father still has 'mental capacity'. This means that he understands what he is doing when he makes a choice. People's mental capacity or competence may change, so it may be possible when seeking consent to choose a time when your father is most alert. The Mental Capacity Act assumes that a person has capacity, so it is necessary to show that your father does not have capacity rather than the other way round.

For a will to be valid, your father will need to be able to understand what a will is, be aware of the size of his estate and be aware of the individuals who may have a claim to the estate. In order to sign a Lasting Power of Attorney, your father also needs to understand, at that time, that he is giving someone the power to manage his personal affairs.

I hold an Enduring Power of Attorney for my mother and I manage her money for her. I have heard about the new Lasting Power of Attorney. Will my Enduring Power still be valid?

Yes, you can continue to use your Enduring Power of Attorney. It covers only financial matters, as you know, so it will not enable you to have the wider role, dealing with living arrangements, health care, treatment and personal care, which a Lasting Power of Attorney provides. If your mother still has mental capacity you may wish to discuss with her giving you these wider responsibilities by making a new Lasting Power of Attorney. You, too, need to consider whether or not you want to do this.

Since the Mental Capacity Act was fully enacted (in October 2007), it is no longer possible to make an Enduring Power of Attorney but those made before the end of September 2007 continue to be valid. A Lasting Power of Attorney allows the person giving the power to choose the areas of control they give to their attorney, so it can be restricted to financial matters only.

I have been diagnosed with dementia and I am worried about being treated against my wishes when I become unable to decide about my health care. I've heard about Living Wills. Should I make one of these?

A Living Will, called an Advance Decision (also known as an Advance Directive), is a document that sets out a person's preferences in their health care and what forms of treatment they would refuse if they were seriously ill and unable to express their wishes. People might wish to object to being fed with a tube, for instance, if they were unable to swallow. An Advance Decision cannot compel a doctor to provide a particular treatment or ask doctors to do anything against the law or against medical ethics. Advance Decisions are binding on a doctor if the doctor knows about them and they are clear in meaning, as well as on anyone holding a Lasting Power of Attorney.

If you decide to make a Living Will, give a copy to your GP for inclusion in your file and make sure that your close relatives or next of kin are aware of its contents.

Suggested forms are available from several organisations, including Dignity in Dying and the Terrence Higgins Trust (contact details in Appendix 1). The Alzheimer's Society also produces a useful fact-sheet and form called 'Advance Decision'.

FINANCIAL CAPACITY

My widowed mother has always been a methodical and well-organised person and doesn't like me to interfere in her financial affairs. However, she is getting forgetful and her electricity was nearly turned off because she hadn't paid the bill. What can I do?

A good way of ensuring that your mother's bills are paid on time would be to suggest that she signs direct debit forms for her utility bills and for any other regular payments, such as rent. If she won't sign a direct debit, perhaps she would find a regular payment by standing order more acceptable.

Most utility companies – water, gas and electricity – have a register of older customers and those with special needs, and you should inform them that your mother may not respond in time. All utility companies will have a code of practice covering any cutting off of the supply, and copies should be available. The various companies will probably agree to inform you if they have a problem with your mother's bills.

You should prepare yourself for the likelihood that your mother's ability to manage her affairs will get worse. Contact the company that supplies your mother, to find out what arrangements they can make.

*My father, who has Alzheimer's disease, is no longer able to
manage his money safely. He forgets to get his pension, loses
cash and refuses to pay for things in shops. What can we do?*

It is usual for people to lose their understanding of money as
Alzheimer's disease progresses. There are a number of practical
things that you can do to keep your father independent for as long as
possible while protecting his money.

One thing you can do is to make arrangements concerning your
father's pension. For example, it may be possible for someone to be
authorised to collect it for him. Contact the local office of the
Department for Work and Pensions (DWP). The person chosen is
known as the 'authorised agent'. However, your father cannot make
a valid choice if he does not understand what he is doing. In this
case, *appointeeship* should be considered. This is a more formal
arrangement and should be made through the Department for Work
and Pensions. Alternatively, if your father has a bank or building
society account, an arrangement can be made for his pension to be
paid directly into that. Ask the Department for Work and Pensions or
your father's bank for advice on how to do this.

If you have an Enduring or Lasting Power of Attorney (see the previous section), you could use it to limit your father's access to cash. If
you don't have a Lasting Power of Attorney (LPA) and it is too late to
get one (see the next answer), you or someone else will need to apply
to become his *receiver*. However, be careful. If you don't have an LPA
or are not a deputy appointed by the Court (see the next answer), the
bank may refuse to deal with you and may take action to freeze your
father's account on the grounds of his mental incapacity. So apply
for an LPA or to be a deputy (see the next answer) before approaching his bank.

If your father is known in the local shops, you may feel able to
explain to the shopkeepers and make arrangements with them to
pay for goods if he refuses to do so. If your father has a helpful bank
or building society manager, it may be wise to speak to them so that
they can alert you if your father takes out more money than he

should need. Many people with dementia lose money. If possible, you should limit the amount of cash that your father has at any time, and should try to ensure that bills and regular payments, such as for gas, electricity, council tax or rent, are paid by standing order or direct debit.

> *My husband has always looked after our money. He used to be so well organised and paid all the bills. He was very unwilling to hand over to me as he became more forgetful. Now he cannot even write a cheque. How can I or our son take over his finances?*

If your husband is able to grant you a Lasting Power of Attorney (LPA; see the previous section), you should take steps to arrange this at once. This is the simplest arrangement.

However, if your husband is not capable of granting a Lasting Power of Attorney, and you live in England or Wales, you will have to apply to the Court of Protection (contact details in Appendix 1) to become his deputy. (Different arrangements apply in Scotland and in Northern Ireland; Alzheimer Scotland or the Alzheimer's Society can advise you on this.)

The Court of Protection is an office of the Supreme Court. It exists to protect the property and finances of people who are mentally unable to manage their own affairs. The Court of Protection will consider the medical evidence about your husband, as well as the details of his financial position and that of his family. Having considered the evidence, the Court then usually appoints a close relative as a *deputy*. If you become your husband's deputy, you will be able to take over his bank account and pay bills and receive income on his behalf as long as you try to act in his best interests. You will be accountable to the Court of Protection for what you do.

Once you have been appointed deputy, the administration is handled by the Public Guardianship Office (contact details in Appendix 1). It will charge a fee when you are appointed deputy and will require you to provide an annual account of how your husband's money has been spent. There will also be an annual fee for administration. Having to go to the Court of Protection to obtain receivership is time-consuming and expensive. Many carers feel very unhappy about this system but it must be remembered that it is designed to protect the person who is mentally incapacitated.

STATE BENEFITS

Are there any financial benefits to help people with Alzheimer's disease?

There are several ways that you can get financial help from the state if you are caring for someone with a dementia such as Alzheimer's disease, although there is no state benefit that relates specifically to people with dementia. The state benefits system can be rather confusing and you may find it helpful to seek advice. Your social worker should be able to help you, or your local Citizens Advice (CAB). There is also a freephone Benefits Enquiry Line (contact details in Appendix 1) for people with disabilities, including people with dementia. The Alzheimer's Society has a useful information sheet on Welfare benefits which provides more detail than can be included here. Also helpful are the Age Concern book *Your Rights to Money Benefits* and the *Disability Benefits Handbook* published by the Disability Alliance, both revised annually.

All state benefits depend in some way on individual financial or personal circumstances. It is best to check out as many different benefits as possible. Some depend on income, others on age and others on the reason, such as illness or unemployment, why help is needed. There is also help available to carers in some situations.

All people with dementia should be able to apply for either Attendance Allowance or Disability Living Allowance to help them with their care needs. These benefits do not depend on income or savings and are tax free. Neither do they take account of where a person lives or if they live alone or with a carer. People whose care needs develop before the age of 65 should apply for Disability Living

Allowance. People aged 65 and over should apply for the Attendance Allowance. Both allowances are paid at different rates depending on the person's needs. The Disability Living Allowance has a mobility payment as well as a care payment.

Either Attendance Allowance or Disability Living Allowance can be paid to people who need help with daily care such as washing, dressing, eating, toileting and taking medication. They can also be paid if people need supervision to avoid risks when inside or outside the home. Because dementia is a progressive illness, it is important to reapply as needs change.

People under the age of 65 who have difficulty walking may apply for the mobility component of the Disability Living Allowance. There are two rates. A lower rate is paid to people who show that, although they are able to walk, they need guidance to stop them getting lost. The higher rate is paid to people who are unable to walk because of paralysis or weakness or whose walking is severely limited. Few people with dementia get the higher rate but it is worth applying, particularly if they also have problems walking. Application forms for the various allowances are available from your local post office or JobCentre Plus. If you need help filling in the forms, your local Alzheimer's Society, carers' group or Citizens Advice may be able to help you.

My husband had to leave his job because he became forgetful and inefficient. He was later diagnosed as having dementia. What financial help can we get? Will his pension rights be affected?

There can be problems for people with dementia who have to give up work or are sacked because of undiagnosed dementia. People may have lost unemployment benefits or sick pay or pension rights. It is important to inform your husband's former employers of the diagnosis and to ask for his rights to be protected. You may have to get medical reports to support your case. Local Alzheimer's Society branches often provide special help for younger people with dementia and have experience of dealing with such problems, so contact them. If your husband was a member of a union or staff association, they may be able to help.

People with dementia who have had to give up work and are below retirement age may be able to apply for Incapacity Benefit. Incapacity Benefit may be claimed if someone is unable to work because of illness or disability and is not entitled to statutory sick pay. The person claiming the benefit must have paid sufficient National Insurance contributions.

If you have given up work to care for your husband, you may be able to apply for Carer's Allowance or for Income Support (see the next answer).

My wife was only 49 when she developed Alzheimer's disease. We managed for a few years on my income after she stopped work. Now I have had to give up working to care for her, so we have very little to live on. Are there any state benefits to help carers?

You should be able to apply for Carers Allowance. This can be paid to carers who spend at least 35 hours a week looking after someone – be they relative, friend or neighbour. The person they look after must be getting either the Attendance Allowance or the Disability Living Allowance at the middle or higher rate. So if your wife is not claiming one of these you should apply for them first.

Carers can claim if they are over 16 years old. Payment does not depend on previous National Insurance contributions. Indeed, this benefit will give you class 1 National Insurance contribution credits to help protect your pension rights when you reach 65. Carers Allowance is taxable. Be aware, though, that receiving Carers Allowance might reduce benefits received by the person you are caring for; it is probably wise to get advice (for example, from a carer's group or Citizens Advice) before applying for it.

If your income is low and your savings are below the limit set by the government, you may also be able to claim Income Support. This is paid to people on low incomes to help them with basic living expenses. Income Support can be paid in full or as a top-up to other benefits or pensions. Attendance Allowance and Disability Living Allowance are ignored as income when calculating Income Support entitlement.

If you are entitled to Income Support, you are also likely to qualify for Housing Benefit and Council Tax Benefit and also for free prescriptions and other NHS benefits. Your social worker or local Citizens Advice should be able to help you work out all the help you and your wife can get.

My mother has come to live with me so that I can care for her. Do I have to pay the full Council Tax now? I used to get the single person's discount.

Your Council Tax is set and collected by your local authority and you should contact them about possible discounts and how to claim them. (People who live in Northern Ireland, where there is still a rating system, should contact the rebate section of the local rate collection agency.) It is likely that you will still qualify for the single person's discount of 25% on your Council Tax bill.

Your mother will be 'disregarded' for the purposes of Council Tax assessment if you are caring for her for at least 35 hours a week and if she is receiving the highest rate of the Disability Living Allowance or Attendance Allowance.

Even if you are still working, you can ask for your mother to be 'disregarded' for Council Tax purposes if she has a medical certificate stating that she is severely mentally impaired and is receiving the Attendance Allowance or the middle rate of the Disability Living Allowance. You may also qualify for a 'disregard' as a carer, which could result in an overall reduction of 50% in your bill.

If your mother still has her own home, it will be exempt from Council Tax while it is empty because she has moved so that you can care for her.

If you need to extend your home by adding an extra room or bathroom because of your mother's disability, you may be able to get a reduction in the Council Tax band. Ask your Council for details of the 'Disability Reduction'.

My husband, who is only 59, has been diagnosed with Alzheimer's disease. Can I get free prescriptions and other help for him?

Your husband has not yet reached the statutory retirement age and so is not entitled to free medical prescriptions on the grounds of age. However, he will qualify for free prescriptions and other NHS benefits if he is receiving Income Support or Disability Living Allowance and has savings of less than the official limit (to check the current limit contact the Benefits Enquiry Line or ask your GP practice). Even if he does not meet these criteria, it might still be worth applying if his income is low.

Other NHS benefits include free dental treatment from NHS dentists, free sight tests and vouchers towards glasses, and free hearing tests and hearing aids. You should also be able to get free continence aids and vouchers for aids such as wheelchairs. Help with travel costs for NHS hospital visits is also available. Ask for claim forms from your husband's GP, the practice nurse or at the hospital.

I have been turned down for the benefit I applied for. How can I appeal?

If you think you have been turned down unfairly for a state benefit, you have a right to disagree with the decision. Write to the office that made the decision and ask them to review it. Give them additional or corrected information if you think they have not taken all the facts into account. If they do not change their decision you may be able to apply to an independent appeal tribunal.

You can also appeal if you think you have not been awarded the correct rate of a benefit, such as the lower or higher rate of the Attendance Allowance or the mobility part of the Disability Living Allowance.

Appealing can be complicated and the rules are different for different benefits, so get advice as soon as possible from a Citizens Advice, your local council Welfare Rights office, the Benefits Enquiry Line, or the Alzheimer's Society or Alzheimer Scotland (contact details in Appendix 1).

My husband went into hospital for an assessment but while he was there he got worse and now it seems unlikely he will be able to come home. What happens to his Attendance Allowance and other benefits?

Your husband's Attendance Allowance will be suspended after he has been in hospital for 28 days. If he has a state retirement pension, this will be reduced after he has been in hospital for six weeks. The amount by which it will be reduced will depend on your husband's actual circumstances. Other benefits, if he is receiving any, may also be affected.

If your husband is discharged from hospital into a care home, new financial arrangements will need to be made. If his fees are to be paid for by the local authority or by the NHS, Attendance Allowance will stop but your husband will be expected to claim all the other benefits he is entitled to. Most of the benefit money will go towards paying the home's fees, but your husband will be entitled to a small sum for personal spending each week. If your husband is paying his own care home fees, he can continue to claim and receive the Attendance Allowance.

OTHER FINANCIAL HELP

My wife has Alzheimer's disease and I have retired early to look after her. Is it possible for us to get grants or financial help from anywhere other than the Department for Work and Pensions?

There are various organisations that may be able to help you with particular bills, items of equipment or respite breaks. Many religious communities offer help to their members. If you or the person you care for belong to a trade union or a benevolent or friendly society, they may be able to help. There are also trusts and charities set up specially to help people connected with the armed forces or who have worked in a particular trade or profession. A number of national and local charities also make small grants to people in need.

Whether you can get help will depend on the rules of the organisation you apply to, what funds are available and what your needs are. You can only find out by making contact with particular organisations.

One directory that might be of use to you is *A Guide to Grants for Individuals in Need*. This lists many sources of help and tells you how to apply. It is published by the Directory of Social Change and should be in your local library.

Your social worker or doctor or local religious group may know about local charities or sources of help.

The national Alzheimer's Society (contact details in Appendix 1) has a dementia support grant. Small grants are available to help with daily living, transport, respite or temporary financial need. An application form is available from the Society. Your local Alzheimer's Society branch may also give small grants or arrange respite breaks.

PAYING FOR CARE HOME FEES

Some people in my area who have dementia are cared for free of charge in hospital, but I have been told I have to find a nursing home for my father. Why do some people get NHS care and others have to go private?

Over the last fifteen years in the UK the number of beds provided by the National Health Service for people with dementia has been greatly reduced. Very few people now receive free care in hospital or through NHS continuing care in a nursing home. Most people who need care in a home pay for themselves or are paid for by the local authority's Social Services Department.

In Scotland 'personal care' is paid for by the state after the person has been assessed by the local authority. Different arrangements apply in England where the NHS will pay only for care provided by a registered nurse (see the section 'Types of homes' in Chapter 10).

There are some people who are entitled to NHS continuing care. Your local Health Authority must publish its criteria for this. These 'eligibility criteria' set out the conditions that must be met if the NHS is to provide or pay for long-term care for someone with dementia. Usually it will only be when a person needs constant nursing care and regular supervision by a hospital consultant by reason of extreme frailty or severe mental disturbance.

If you look at the eligibility criteria in your area and think that your father meets them, you can ask his consultant to admit him to an NHS bed, or simply ask for him to be assessed for NHS continuing care. If the hospital won't accept him, you can ask for a review. However, the review will look only at whether the eligibility criteria have been properly applied, not at whether they are fair in the first place. The Alzheimer's Society Helpline (see Appendix 1) provides information about NHS continuing care.

My mother has fairly substantial savings but does not own her own home. She gets the state widow's pension. Will she have to pay for all her nursing home care?

Your mother will have to pay for her own nursing home care if she has savings of more than the official limit (in 2007 the savings limit was between £20,000 and £22,000, depending on which UK country you lived in). Her state widow's pension is unlikely to cover more than a small proportion of the fees, so she will have to find the rest of the money from her savings.

If your mother has enough money to pay for nursing home fees for the foreseeable future, you and she can make your own choice of home and financial arrangements. However, if you choose a luxurious and expensive home, your mother will probably have to move to a cheaper home approved by Social Services if her money ever runs out.

If you think that your mother's savings are not likely to cover her home fees indefinitely, ask Social Services to conduct an assessment of her needs (see the section 'Community care' in Chapter 9) *before* you find her a home. If the assessment confirms that your mother does need to go into a nursing home, they will then do a nursing needs assessment (see the section 'Types of homes' in Chapter 10) to see how much the NHS will contribute to the cost of her care. Social Services will specify the amount that they will pay as and when your mother's savings are reduced to below the official limit.

If you do not get an assessment of her needs before your mother goes into a home, check whether the home's fees fall within Social Services' limits. If they do, you should make arrangements with your GP or Social Services to assess your mother's needs well before her savings fall to the level that will qualify her for financial help from the local authority.

Social Services are arranging for my wife to be moved into a nursing home. They are making a financial assessment of her income and savings and have asked me to tell them about my money as well. Is this right?

The local authority can assess only the financial resources of the person who is receiving care. They do not have the power to insist that you provide details of your income or savings. The local authority has to work out your wife's contribution to her care costs based on her finances. They have a duty to make up the difference, if any, between the cost of the nursing home and her contribution.

However, the 1948 National Assistance Act (section 42) states that husbands and wives are liable to support each other financially. This is one of the 'liable relative rules' and applies to married couples and to civil partners under the Civil Partnerships Act 2004. Your local authority can ask you to make a contribution but has no power to insist that you reveal details of your finances to them. Normally, a husband or wife can make an offer of an amount that he or she thinks is reasonable to pay towards the cost of caring for their spouse.

> *I have cared for my husband, who has Alzheimer's disease, for a number of years now but recently I have been ill myself and we have reluctantly decided that he should go into a nursing home. He has an occupational pension as well as his state retirement pension, and we have savings of about £50,000. It seems that he will have to pay his own care home fees but this leaves me with very little to live on. Is there anything I can do?*

It can be very hard on the partner when a husband or wife goes into a nursing home and pays their own fees out of what was previously shared income and savings.

Your husband will pay his own fees until his share of your joint savings is reduced to the official limit.

You may find, if you do the sums, that splitting your savings in half and keeping them in separate accounts will allow you to keep more of your money. You will continue to receive the married woman's pension. You may also claim half of your husband's occupational pension. If this is a very small amount, however, you may be better off not claiming it and applying for Income Support instead. If you receive Income Support, you will also be able to get Housing Benefit and various NHS benefits (for more information, see the section 'State benefits' earlier in this chapter) when your savings are below the official limit.

My husband has become incontinent and I really can't cope with looking after him any more. It seems that a nursing home is the only choice now but he only has a small pension. Will I have to sell our house to pay the home's fees? And what money will I have to live on?

You will not have to sell the house while you continue to live in it. You should ask your GP or Social Services to carry out a needs assessment (see the section 'Types of homes' in Chapter 10). If your husband is considered to need a nursing home, you can choose a home from the list which Social Services should give you. Social Services will make arrangements to pay your husband's fees direct to the home. The Health Service will contribute in three payment bands towards the cost of his nursing care (see 'Types of homes' in Chapter 10). Recent changes to the banding system mean that, for people who enter a home after 1 October 2007, care homes will receive a flat rate of £101 per week, regardless of the level of nursing care required. If you have your own state pension, all of his state pension will go towards the cost of the nursing home. If your husband has an occupational pension, you can claim half of that. If he has no occupational pension and you have no pension of your own, you will be left with only the married woman's pension, which is not much to live on. You may be entitled to Income Support.

While you live in the house, Social Services will not ask you to sell it to pay for your husband's fees. However, if you stop living in it because you move or you die, they can make a claim against the proceeds of the sale. If your husband alone owns the house, all the value will be taken into account. If it is owned jointly, half of it will be considered his.

I moved in with my father after my mother died. I have cared for him for many years but now he has had to go into a nursing home. I always thought that the house would be mine. It is left to me in his will but now it seems that Social Services will take it to pay for his care. Is this right?

All your father's income and savings and assets (usually including the house) over the official limit will be taken into account, after a period of three months, when Social Services work out how much he has to contribute to the cost of the nursing home. Social Services may disregard the value of the house in some circumstances and you should ask them if they are willing to do so. In certain circumstances they must disregard it, for instance if the relative living in it is over 60 years old or is disabled.

As long as you continue to live in the house, Social Services are unlikely to take it from you or sell it. They can apply for a court order to force you to sell the house but this is very rare. If you remain in the house, they may later 'make a charge' against it (require repayment) for whatever amount they have contributed to your father's nursing home costs. This amount will be payable only if you decide to move and sell the house. When your father dies, the house will be yours but there may still be a charge against your father's estate if you decide to sell it.

12 | Treatment

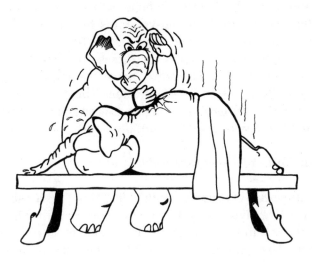

Although there is no cure for Alzheimer's disease or for most other types of dementia, it is possible to help people with dementia, and their carers, in a variety of ways. Many of the problems associated with dementia, such as restlessness and depression, can be treated. It may also be possible, especially in the early stages of dementia, to improve someone's memory with medication or by using other methods. People with dementia may also develop other, unrelated, illnesses that require treatment.

TREATMENT POSSIBILITIES

Is there a cure for Alzheimer's disease?

Unfortunately, there is no cure for Alzheimer's disease at the present time. Nor can a cure be expected in the foreseeable future.

However, in recent years there has been significant progress in the development of drugs (see 'Drug treatments' later in this chapter) that alleviate some of the symptoms of Alzheimer's disease, such as poor memory and the changes in behaviour that occur in the later stages of dementia (see 'Treating symptoms' later in this chapter).

These developments go some way to lessen the symptoms in some people but they do not reverse the disease process or 'cure' Alzheimer's disease. It is still not known how to prevent the disease from occurring or how to stop its progression. There is a great deal of research into the causes of Alzheimer's disease going on throughout the world and the hope is that eventually a cure may be possible.

Are any forms of dementia curable?

Some rare forms of dementia – including those associated with an under-active thyroid gland, brain tumours, or some vitamin deficiencies (for example, of vitamin B_{12}) – can be cured, or helped considerably, by appropriate treatment. Sometimes this treatment is simple, such as taking tablets of thyroid hormone to treat dementia caused by under-activity of the thyroid gland.

Most types of dementia, however, cannot be cured and those that can be are very rare. Nevertheless, it is important not to miss curable causes of dementia and this is one reason why everyone suspected of having dementia should be properly assessed by a doctor.

There is no scientific evidence that taking thyroid hormone or vitamin supplements is helpful for people with dementia who do not have a deficiency in these substances. Indeed, the inappropriate use of such supplements can sometimes be harmful.

I get so frustrated. I keep coming across stories about new treatments for Alzheimer's disease, but nothing seems to be available for my wife. Why is this?

It is very frustrating to read or hear about new treatments only to find out later that they are not actually available. This is especially true when someone, like you, has a personal reason for hoping that a cure may soon be found.

The best advice is to treat all media reports with caution. Millions of people in the world want news of treatments for Alzheimer's disease. When scientists find a treatment that shows promise, they often publicise this widely. This publicity is often premature, as it takes something like ten years between the finding of a new treatment and its availability to the public, during which time the treatment's effectiveness and safety are tested rigorously (for information about testing, see the section 'Drug trials' in Chapter 13). All too often, this later research finds that a treatment that initially looked promising does not work or has dangerous side effects.

For the most up-to-date information on new treatment, you could contact the Alzheimer's Society (address in Appendix 1) or look at reliable sites on the internet (see 'Research overview' in Chapter 13 and website details in Appendix 1).

New drugs for treating Alzheimer's disease have attracted a lot of publicity recently. These drugs have been found to relieve some of the symptoms of Alzheimer's disease and some other types of dementia. However, they are not a cure. They are best taken early in the course of the disease and may not help everyone. These drugs should be available to your wife on the NHS and you should see your doctor about this. (See also the section 'Drug treatments' later in this chapter.)

Can anything halt or slow down the mental deterioration that occurs in Alzheimer's disease?

Alzheimer's disease is progressive, leading to death between five and ten years after diagnosis in most cases. However, it may be possible to slow down the rate at which the disease progresses. One possibility is the use of one of the new dementia drugs (see 'Drug treatments' later in this chapter).

The progression of Alzheimer's disease also may be slowed if good general health can be maintained. A well-balanced diet and regular exercise are important. Various simple measures may also contribute by helping to protect the brain, such as not drinking excessive quantities of alcohol, not smoking and avoiding head injuries. It makes good sense to keep all these risks to a minimum when somebody already has dementia. On the other hand, if someone has been a smoker and derives considerable pleasure from this, it may be kinder to allow them to continue to smoke (safely) while they still enjoy it and ask for cigarettes.

A person's physical surroundings are also important – keeping their environment safe and familiar will help to reduce confusion and may reduce the risk of falls.

My wife has vascular dementia. Can anything help to stop things getting worse?

It may be possible to slow down the development of vascular dementia (see the section 'Types of dementia' in Chapter 1) by treating the underlying problem, which is usually cerebrovascular disease (narrowing of the arteries causing reduced blood supply to the brain).

Smoking is known to thicken the blood and to increase the risk of having a stroke. Any smoker who has been given a diagnosis of vascular dementia should seriously consider giving up smoking.

In some cases, the doctor will prescribe drugs, such as aspirin, to thin the blood and decrease the risk of stroke. Any irregularity of the heartbeat should also be treated, as this condition also increases the risk of stroke. People with this condition may also be prescribed warfarin, which is very good at thinning the blood, but needs careful monitoring.

If the arteries leading to the brain have become furred up by sticky deposits (known as 'plaques'), it may be possible to perform an operation to strip away the plaques, thus widening the diameter of the artery and improving the blood supply to the brain. However, this operation has risks and is appropriate only in special circumstances. Your wife's doctor will advise you if the operation might be suitable for her.

If your wife's vascular dementia is accompanied by high blood pressure, this will need careful treatment. A person with cerebrovascular disease may need a relatively high blood pressure to ensure that there is an adequate supply of blood to the brain. However, if the blood pressure is very high, it can cause serious problems and will definitely need to be treated.

Some of the drugs (e.g. galantamine/Reminyl) that have been developed for the treatment of Alzheimer's disease have also been found to be of some help in vascular dementia. Although current recommendations by the National Institute for Health and Clinical Excellence (NICE) limit the use of these drugs to people with Alzheimer's disease, some doctors do prescribe them for other forms of dementia such as vascular dementia. (See 'Drug treatments' later in this chapter for more about new drugs and NICE.)

DEALING WITH DOCTORS

As the carer doing all the work, I feel I should be kept fully informed about my father's illness. But my father's doctor says he is bound by confidentiality and cannot discuss the details with me.

It is true that a doctor's relationship is directly with his or her patient and technically there is a duty of confidentiality between doctor and patient. However, when the person who is ill is not able to understand what is happening to them, doctors usually recognise the need to involve the carer in discussions and decisions. Many doctors now see that it is essential to involve carers in discussions about the diagnosis and care of a patient. Furthermore, if a patient is not able to give consent, the doctor has a duty to act in the patient's best interest and this almost certainly will include discussing things with you, as your father's carer. If you have not already done so, try to explain to your father's doctor how important it is for you to know what is going on. If the doctor is still unwilling to involve you, there are a number of things you can do:

- Ask your father if you can stay with him when he sees the doctor. If your father consents to your being there, the doctor will probably not refuse.

- If it is your father's hospital specialist who is being uncommunicative, try talking about the problem with the GP, or vice versa.

- Talk this through with other carers, or the Alzheimer's Society, as they may have some helpful suggestions.

- Try to talk to other health professionals, such as the practice nurse or the community mental health nurse.

- If all else fails, you could consider changing your father's doctor.

The Mental Capacity Act 2005 allows people in England and Wales to set up a Lasting Power of Attorney, giving someone the authority to make care decisions on their behalf. This person – the 'attorney' – will have the right to talk to doctors and to be involved in decisions about the care of the person they are acting for. The Lasting Power of Attorney has to be set up while someone has 'mental capacity' (see the section 'Legal safeguards' in Chapter 11).

The law is different in Scotland (see Chapter 11).

My mother, who is in a nursing home because of dementia, has been put on sedative drugs. I'm not happy with this. Shouldn't I have been consulted?

Yes, ideally you should have been consulted, although the doctor is under no obligation to talk to you beforehand unless you hold your mother's Lasting Power of Attorney (see the section 'Legal safeguards' in Chapter 11). Sometimes medication is needed to reduce anxiety or difficult behaviour in people with dementia, and modern, non-sedating drug treatments may be appropriate for your mother. However, the home should try to keep you informed of any changes to your mother's treatment.

You may find it helpful to let the staff at the home know that you want to continue to be involved in decisions about your mother's care. If you are unhappy about your mother's treatment, ask the manager of the home to make an appointment for you to see the home's doctor.

SEEING A SPECIALIST

My husband has recently been diagnosed as having Alzheimer's disease. The diagnosis was made by our GP. Should my husband now see a specialist?

General practitioners (GPs) can often diagnose dementia without needing to refer the patient to a specialist. It is usual for GPs to refer a patient on to a specialist if they are not sure about the diagnosis, if the patient might be suitable for treatment with dementia drugs or if they think that the case is not clear-cut.

If the GP does decide to ask for a second opinion, he or she may request this from a geriatrician (a doctor who specialises in physical illnesses in older people) or from a psychiatrist with a particular interest in the mental problems of older people. The GP may occasionally refer someone with dementia to a psychologist (a specialist in mental processes, such as memory) or a neurologist (a doctor who specialises in diseases of the nervous system).

A GP is able to refer people to Social Services for a needs assessment so that they can receive appropriate care and support from the local authority. However, some Social Services departments require the opinion of a specialist before they will proceed. Your husband's GP will know what is necessary in your area. (See Chapter 9 for more information about assessments and community care.)

DRUG TREATMENTS

If drugs can't cure Alzheimer's disease, what can they do for someone who has it?

It is true that, as yet, no drugs have been discovered that can cure Alzheimer's disease or stop it from getting worse over time. However, some dementia drugs are now available that may improve some of the symptoms such as memory loss and disorientation, and can slow down the progression of the symptoms (see the other answers in this section for more information).

Other kinds of drugs are sometimes useful for treating some of the changes in behaviour, such as sleeplessness and agitation, that occur with dementia.

In general, the use of drugs such as sleeping pills or tranquillisers (sedatives) should be kept to a minimum if someone has Alzheimer's disease, as they can cause increased confusion and falls (see the section 'Treating symptoms' later in this chapter).

A person with Alzheimer's disease may need drugs to treat other illnesses that might develop, such as a chest infection, or longer-term medical conditions, such as high blood pressure or diabetes.

My father is taking various kinds of pills, but he seems to be getting more and more confused. Might the drugs he is taking be making his Alzheimer's disease worse rather than better?

It is possible that some of your father's pills may be making him more confused; for example, drugs used for treating all sorts of conditions such as high blood pressure or pain can cause confusion as a side effect. If you tell your father's doctor about your worry, he or she may be able to improve matters by adjusting your father's medication.

In general, it is best for people with Alzheimer's disease to take as few drugs as possible, because certain types of drugs do have side effects that can make confusion worse. Drugs that can cause confusion include tranquillising medication and some painkillers, which may sometimes need to be given to people with dementia.

I have heard that there are some drug treatments for Alzheimer's disease. What are these drugs ?

In the past decade there have been significant advances in the treatment of Alzheimer's disease, and hopefully other dementias. The main development has been the introduction of two types of drugs.

The first type is called *cholinesterase inhibitors* or *anticholinesterase drugs*. These drugs reduce the breakdown of acetylcholine, a chemical found in the brain. Anticholinesterase drugs currently available in the UK include donepezil (Aricept), galantamine (Reminyl) and rivastigmine (Exelon).

The second type of drug is the *NMDA antagonists*. NMDA stands for N-methyl-D-aspartate, one of the chemicals involved in memory. At present one drug of this type is available, called memantine (Ebixa).

These drugs are discussed in later answers in this section.

How do the dementia drugs help people with Alzheimer's disease?

Several clinical trials have found that anticholinesterase drugs seem to relieve some of the symptoms of Alzheimer's disease in some people. People who take these drugs may experience a slight improvement, but the main effect is that the drugs delay worsening of the symptoms of dementia – in some people by up to six months, or even longer. These drugs do not work in all patients and their effect is variable. There is no certainty about how long these drugs will continue to be useful. If they do help someone, their effect can be expected to last from a few months to a year or more. At the moment it is not possible to predict which people will be helped by these drugs.

Although anticholinesterase drugs may help to slow the progress of symptoms in some people, they cannot halt the disease altogether nor reverse any brain damage that has already taken place. These drugs are more likely to help people in the early stage of Alzheimer's disease than to benefit those who already have severe dementia.

Why does the same drug have different names?

Most drugs have two names: a generic name (without a capital first letter) and a brand name (with a capital letter). The *generic* name is the official medical name for the basic active ingredient (e.g. donepezil) and is chosen by the British Pharmacopoeia Commission. The *brand name* (e.g. Aricept) is a name selected by the company that produces the drug. Different manufacturers give different names to the same generic drug in order to differentiate their product. Whatever the name on the box or bottle, the medicine inside will be the same as the one the doctor has prescribed.

How do the new drugs for treating dementia work?

To date, the most promising new drugs belong to a group of dementia drugs called cholinesterase inhibitors or anticholinesterase drugs. Drugs of this type work by reducing the breakdown of acetylcholine in the brain.

Acetylcholine is a chemical that occurs naturally in the brain, where it is continually being made and broken down. Acetylcholine is a 'neurotransmitter' – a chemical that enables nerve cells in the brain to pass messages to each other. In a normal brain, the total level of acetylcholine remains fairly constant. Research has found, however, that the brains of many people with Alzheimer's disease have a reduced amount of acetylcholine, and it is thought that the loss of this chemical may result in deterioration of memory.

Much of the research so far carried out into finding ways of correcting acetylcholine deficiency in the brains of people with Alzheimer's disease has been directed towards increasing the amount of acetylcholine. However, the evidence seems to suggest that giving people this chemical directly does not help. The alternative approach of reducing the rate at which acetylcholine is broken down currently seems more promising, and has resulted so far in the development of three cholinesterase-inhibiting drugs: donepezil (Aricept), galantamine (Reminyl) and rivastigmine (Exelon).

As well as reducing the breakdown of acetylcholine in the brain, galantamine (Reminyl) has another action. It directly stimulates areas in the brain called nicotinic receptors. These receptors may also be involved in memory and learning. It is not clear yet whether this dual action is more effective than the action of other available dementia drugs.

My wife has been diagnosed with Alzheimer's disease but our doctor won't prescribe Aricept. Is there anything I can do about this?

There are several reasons why your doctor may not prescribe Aricept (the brand name of donepezil) or any of the other new drugs mentioned earlier for treating dementia. One possibility is that your wife's Alzheimer's disease is already too advanced, as this treatment is probably less helpful for people with severe dementia. Another possibility is that your wife does not actually have Alzheimer's disease but has another form of dementia – such as vascular dementia (see the section 'Types of dementia' in Chapter 1); some doctors refer to all types of dementia as 'Alzheimer's disease'. There isn't enough research at the moment to convince all doctors that these drugs help vascular dementia. Or your wife may be on other treatments, or have other medical conditions which mean that she shouldn't receive these drugs. Also, some doctors are not convinced that these drugs are effective and are reluctant to prescribe them to anyone. You may wish to ask for a second opinion.

At present in the UK only specialists (psychiatrists, neurologists, geriatricians) can start the prescription of dementia drugs, although their use can be continued by a GP. If your wife has not seen a specialist, you should ask your GP to refer her for a second opinion. If it is the specialist who is unwilling to prescribe the drugs, you can ask your GP to refer your wife to a different specialist. In any event, it may be helpful just to talk with the doctor about his or her reason for not prescribing a dementia drug.

I recently read that NICE has said that drug treatments for dementia should be restricted. Is this true?

The National Institute for Health and Clinical Excellence (NICE) was set up by the UK government to provide recommendations and guidance on a variety of new treatments.

In November 2006 NICE produced guidance on the use of the dementia drugs donepezil (Aricept), galantamine (Reminyl) and rivastigmine (Exelon). NICE recommended that the use of these drugs should be restricted to people with Alzheimer's disease (as opposed to any other dementia), and that the diagnosis must have been made by a specialist. To qualify, a person should also score between 20 and 10 on the Mini Mental State Examination (a short test of memory and concentration used by doctors and nurses; see 'Memory tests' in Chapter 3). This means that these drugs are restricted to people with moderate Alzheimer's disease and doctors are advised not to prescribe them in the early stages of the disease. NICE also recommended that memantine (Ebixa) is not prescribed at all.

Not all doctors, or other groups who are involved in advocating for people with dementia, agree with these guidelines from NICE, and the guidance is not binding on doctors. However, in many areas, funding for the drugs is likely to be restricted to patients who meet the criteria set out by NICE, so people with mild dementia may not be able to have them prescribed.

Are drugs such as Aricept, Exelon, Reminyl and Ebixa effective for everyone with Alzheimer's disease?

These drugs seem to help some, but by no means all, people with Alzheimer's disease. Even if they are effective, they go only some way towards reducing memory problems and other difficulties. Some people may have a significant benefit. However, with many people there is only a minimal benefit or no response at all.

Unfortunately, it is not possible to tell in advance who will respond well to this type of treatment. The effectiveness of the drug does not seem to be affected by the patient's age, sex or ethnic origin. It is less clear whether these drugs are useful in other types of dementia, although there is some promising evidence they may be (see the next answer). Ebixa (memantine) may be more useful in people with more advanced dementia.

At the moment the only way to find out whether a drug is effective is to try it for a few months. If someone gets noticeably worse soon after starting one of these drugs, it is probably not working.

Are the new treatments for Alzheimer's disease helpful for people with other types of dementia?

They may be. For example, rivastigmine (Exelon) has helped people with Lewy body dementia and galantamine (Reminyl) may also help in vascular dementia (see 'Types of dementia' in Chapter 1). The likelihood is that these drugs may help in all the common types of dementia (Alzheimer's disease, vascular dementia and Lewy body dementia), though they don't work for everyone. Although the NICE guidelines (see earlier answers) say that the drugs donepezil (Aricept) etc. should be used only for Alzheimer's disease, some specialists are prescribing these drugs for other types of dementia.

Do dementia drugs, such as Aricept, have side effects?

Any drug may cause side effects and sometimes these are unpredictable and unpleasant. The main side effects of dementia drugs include nausea, vomiting and diarrhoea. However, most people are able to tolerate the side effects and continue the medication. Side effects vary from drug to drug and from person to person but tend to become less troublesome after a few weeks.

My wife tried Exelon but the doctor stopped it because she got bad side effects. Is it worth trying another dementia drug?

It may be. If rivastigmine (Exelon) was stopped because it wasn't working, it is unlikely that another drug of the same type would be any better. However, in your wife's case, the drug was stopped because of side effects. Side effects do differ from drug to drug and it may be worth trying another one such as donepezil (Aricept) or galantamine (Reminyl). You and your wife should speak to your wife's doctor.

I have been taking Reminyl for six months and it seems to suit me. I have heard that another drug, Ebixa, is now available. Should I take this as well?

Ebixa (memantine) works in a different way from the cholinesterase inhibitors such as donepezil (Aricept), galantamine (Reminyl) or rivastigmine (Exelon). It is not clear whether taking Ebixa together with one of these other drugs will add any benefit, and it may cause more side effects. It is probably better to just stick to the drug you are on.

My aunt recently started on Aricept and seems a little better. How long can I expect this effect to last?

It is quite common for someone to respond to a dementia drug, such as donepezil (Aricept) or rivastigmine (Exelon), within the first few weeks of starting to take it. The drug won't stop your aunt from getting worse but it may slow down the rate at which this happens. It is not clear how long the effects of the dementia drug will last but clinical trials up to one year in length suggest that, if someone does respond to a dementia drug, the improvement may be sustained for at least a year. Other research suggests that the effect may last over three years in some people. A possible problem with these drugs is that, once someone stops taking the drug, their memory may deteriorate more rapidly, so they may soon find themselves in the position they would have been in if they had never taken the drug at all. So, if your aunt seems better on Aricept, it may be best for her to stay on it as long as possible.

TREATING SYMPTOMS

My husband, who has Alzheimer's, sleeps very little and is very restless at night. This disturbs my sleep too and I am getting very tired. Could he take sleeping pills, or might they make him more confused?

The decision to give sleeping pills to someone with Alzheimer's disease should not be taken lightly. Sedatives, such as sleeping pills and tranquillisers, can increase confusion. They can also cause unsteadiness of gait, which may lead to falls. It is therefore wise to avoid them if at all possible.

Possible alternatives to sleeping pills may include practical measures, such as providing plenty of activity during the day (see Chapter 5 for ideas), preventing too many cat-naps, avoiding caffeine, especially in the evening, not giving a heavy meal late at night, giving a relaxing bath before bed and making sure that the bedroom is warm and comfortable.

In some circumstances, however, the use of sleeping pills or tranquillisers may be necessary. Some 'tranquillisers' are not sedative, that is they do not cause excessive sleepiness but can help to ensure a full night's sleep. You should discuss this with your husband's doctor if you are worried.

You say that you are getting very tired. In view of this, it would probably be sensible to talk to your doctor about the possibility of sleeping pills for your husband, at least for a time, or seeing whether Social Services can provide some respite care. (Chapter 9 has more information about getting help.)

My mother's dementia seems to be getting worse and she often becomes very agitated and upset. I used to be able to distract or calm her myself, but she no longer responds to my efforts. Might drugs help?

As well as confusion, anybody with dementia can develop other symptoms, including anxiety, depression, agitation, aggressiveness, strange beliefs and hallucinations. These symptoms are very common and many people with dementia experience them at some point.

In general, doctors try if possible to avoid using drugs to treat anxiety and agitation in people with Alzheimer's disease. Drugs such as tranquillisers can have side effects that outweigh their benefits.

The first thing to do is to make sure that there is not another reason for your mother becoming agitated or upset. Simple things such as pain or constipation can cause agitation and your mother may not be able to tell you what is happening. Certainly it is important that your mother has a check-up to make sure that there is not another cause for this. One possibility might be for your mother's doctor to involve a clinical psychologist who has experience of working with people with dementia. He or she may be able to offer you useful advice on how to carry on managing your mother.

In some cases, especially in the later stages of Alzheimer's disease, tranquillisers may be the best option for increasing the quality of life both for people with dementia and for their carers. Research has shown that some of the newer tranquillisers, such as risperidone or olanzapine, may have a calming effect without causing excessive sedation or other side effects such as stiffness or shaking. However, these should be used for short periods only and it has recently been suggested that these drugs may increase the risk of stroke in people with dementia. This is something you should talk through with your mother's doctor because the risks of taking drugs such as risperidone often outweigh the benefits.

There are other drugs that may be able to help, such as carbamazepine (normally used in epilepsy but have been found to be effective in this situation). It is fair to say that, currently, drugs should be used only as a last resort.

The best approach is to talk this through with your mother's doctor. He or she may want to refer your mother to a specialist for further advice. If your mother is started on a tranquilliser, make sure that the need for this drug is reviewed regularly, as she may not need it for more than a few months. We deal with other ways of helping with agitation and distress in Chapter 7.

I understand that constipation can cause increased agitation in people with Alzheimer's disease. Might laxative drugs be useful?

It is true that constipation can cause increased agitation in people with Alzheimer's disease. In the first instance, constipation is best treated by dietary measures. More bran, fruit and vegetables will often help to ease the problem. Some people may find such foods difficult to accept, but others seem to thrive on them. Drinking plenty of fluids during the day, and regular exercise when possible, should also help.

It is recognised, however, that further treatment is needed in some cases. A doctor will be able to give advice on the possible use of laxatives, such as ispaghula (e.g. Regulan, Fybogel) and lactulose. In some cases, where poor co-ordination and weak anal sphincter muscles are factors, a regular enema may be the best treatment.

I've heard that giving tranquillisers can make people with Alzheimer's disease worse. Is this true?

There is always a risk when taking any sort of medication but this should be balanced in each case against the potential benefits. Tranquillisers are no exception.

There are many types of tranquillisers that may be used and each has its own potential problems. Two groups are in common use: drugs called *benzodiazepines* (such as diazepam (Valium) or temazepam) and drugs known as *antipsychotics* (such as olanzapine, quetiapine and risperidone). All tranquillisers can make people sleepy and more confused during the day. Before prescribing tranquillisers, the doctor should assess the person's physical condition (including blood pressure and heart rhythm) and carefully weigh up the benefits and side effects.

The point of giving tranquillisers is to calm someone down if they are agitated, or to give them a restful night's sleep if they would otherwise be up and about disturbing not only themselves but also carers and other family members. However, tranquillisers can reduce co-ordination, resulting in falls. This is particularly a problem in older people, who may not be able to get up easily off the floor, even with the help of a carer. Furthermore, older people with fragile bones may sustain a fracture if they fall. For these reasons it is always important to make sure that the dose of tranquilliser is correct: not too little so that it doesn't work and not too much so that it makes people drowsy or uncoordinated. If you are worried about someone you care for being given tranquillisers, you should talk to his or her doctor.

Some tranquillising medication (known as antipsychotic drugs or neuroleptic drugs) may occasionally cause side effects that make people more restless rather than less. If someone starts taking these tablets and seems more restless as a result, you should let the doctor know so that the dose can be reduced or the tablets stopped altogether. These drugs may also increase the risk of stroke in people with dementia and are best prescribed under specialist supervision.

Our doctor has prescribed temazepam to help my husband sleep. I gather this medicine is similar to Valium. Is it addictive?

Temazepam and diazepam (Valium) are commonly used tranquillisers that can be very useful for calming people who are agitated and helping them to get to sleep. Tranquillisers of this type may cause dependence (a form of addiction) in some people. This means that it can be difficult to stop these tablets, and doing so may cause withdrawal symptoms, notably feeling unwell or anxious.

Generally speaking, addiction is a problem only if these drugs are taken for three weeks or more. If you are worried about your husband becoming addicted, talk to your doctor. Sometimes the risks of addiction are outweighed by the benefits of the medication. Alternatively, there are other medicines, such as zopiclone (Zimovane), that help sleep and are possibly less addictive. Sometimes, general measures, such as avoiding caffeine and having a relaxing bath before bed, may be enough.

Other medicines your doctor may prescribe, including drugs known as neuroleptics (or antipsychotics) and antidepressants, are not addictive. Don't be afraid to discuss with the doctor any medications that are prescribed.

My wife, who has Alzheimer's, seems to be suffering from hallucinations, which sometimes make her very distressed. Can anything be done to help?

Hallucinations – in which a person sees, hears, smells or feels something when there is nothing there to cause it – are fairly common in people with Alzheimer's disease and other types of dementia. The tendency to experience them varies, not only from day to day but also over time. Sometimes, hallucinations, especially visual hallucinations, are worse at night or in poor lighting, when people are more likely to misinterpret what they see. If someone becomes more agitated at night, the occurrence of hallucinations should be considered as a possibility. In many people, hallucinations seem to stop occurring as the disease progresses.

Treatment of hallucinations in people with Alzheimer's disease should begin with trying to reassure them that what they are experiencing is not really happening. If your wife is very distressed and will not accept this reassurance, her doctor may have to resort to medication that can help to reduce the hallucinations. Small doses of the newer tranquillisers may result in a substantial reduction in the hallucinations without significant side effects. However, your wife's doctor will need to weigh up carefully the potential benefit of giving these drugs to your wife against their potential side effects, which include worsening confusion and possibly increasing the risk of stroke.

Hallucinations are very common in people with other types of dementia such as Lewy body dementia and dementia associated with Parkinson's disease (see the section 'Types of dementia' in Chapter 1). If people with these types of dementia are given antipsychotic drugs, they can get very bad side effects and for this reason it is best for them not to have these drugs. However, dementia drugs such as rivastigmine (Exelon) may be helpful.

Is there any point in treating other mental health conditions, such as depression and anxiety, in someone who has been diagnosed with Alzheimer's disease?

During the course of a dementia such as Alzheimer's disease, treatment may be needed for a variety of physical and mental disorders. It is very important always to get appropriate treatment for physical illnesses when someone has Alzheimer's disease, because quite minor illnesses can produce either worsening of the dementia or acute confusion. Many underlying medical illnesses can be treated.

Depression is relatively common in older people, and more common with dementia. Scientists estimate that as many as four in ten people with dementia will become depressed at some point. Some people with Alzheimer's disease will have had recurring bouts of depression before developing the dementia. Others will be experiencing a depressive illness for the first time. Given that depression can lead to failure to eat and drink, causing severe weight loss, unexplained behaviour problems and sheer misery, it certainly merits treatment. (See the next answer for more information.)

Anxiety frequently accompanies the early stages of a dementia and, at this stage, is usually best dealt with by reassurance rather than drug therapy. Later, when reassurance is more difficult, and in people who suffer from long-term anxiety disorder, medication can be useful.

How do you treat someone who has depression and dementia?

The two mainstays of treatment for depression are medication and 'talking therapies' (psychotherapy and cognitive therapy). Both may sometimes have a role in the treatment of depression in a person with dementia.

In someone with quite an advanced dementia, however, talking therapies are not usually possible because the person is too confused and cannot concentrate for long enough. Furthermore, these treatments are sometimes not easily obtainable and can be expensive. For these reasons, many doctors resort to medication in the first instance.

There are several different types of antidepressant tablets. Some of the older antidepressants are possibly best avoided because they may cause side effects that make memory problems worse. Some newer antidepressants, such as those belonging to the group known as serotonin specific reuptake inhibitors (SSRIs), for example paroxetine and citalopram, do not have these side effects.

It is often difficult to be sure whether someone with a dementia such as Alzheimer's disease is also experiencing depression. In view of this, a doctor may decide to prescribe a course of antidepressant tablets and see what happens. The tablets will have to be taken regularly for at least two weeks before there is any obvious effect. The signs of an improvement can be quite subtle, perhaps just less agitation and a more cheerful disposition. In some cases, there are also improvements in memory. It is important, however, not to be too optimistic about any such improvements in memory. The dementia itself does not respond to treatment with antidepressant drugs.

SURGERY

We have been told that my husband has Alzheimer's disease.
Would an operation on his brain help?

At present there is no operation that can help people with Alzheimer's disease. On the contrary, there is a risk that any type of operation will make a person with Alzheimer's disease more confused.

One very rare form of dementia, called 'normal pressure hydrocephalus' (discussed in the section 'Types of dementia' in Chapter 1), may possibly be helped by an operation to drain fluid from the brain. Diagnosis of normal pressure hydrocephalus can be difficult, but it is extremely unlikely that your husband has this condition rather than Alzheimer's disease. Also, even if someone does have normal pressure hydrocephalus, an operation is not always advised.

My husband, who has recently been diagnosed with Alzheimer's
disease, has finally been offered a long-awaited hip-replacement
operation. Should he have the operation or might it make his
confusion worse?

People with dementia should have appropriate treatment for physical illnesses, and this sometimes includes operations. However, someone with Alzheimer's disease can find going into hospital very confusing and the use of anaesthetics and pain-relieving drugs may temporarily increase confusion. There is also a risk that the confusion will be permanently worse after the operation. This risk needs to be balanced against the potential benefits of having the hip replacement.

Whether it is a good idea for your husband to have his hip-replacement operation will depend on the details of his case, such as how much pain he is experiencing and how severe his dementia is. It may be possible, for example, for the surgeon to do the operation using a spinal, rather than general, anaesthetic. In view of this, your best action would be to discuss the situation with the orthopaedic staff at the hospital, so that a proper assessment of risks and benefits can be made.

PSYCHOLOGICAL TREATMENTS

What is involved in reminiscence therapy? And is it useful for people with dementia?

Reminiscence therapy involves stimulating the recollection of events or memories from the past. This is achieved by using music, videotapes or pictures (for example, films of trams or photographs of early cinema idols) or by providing articles such as food packaging or items of clothing from past eras. It may work because people's memories for events from the distant past are often better than more recent memories. Reminiscence therapy is usually carried out in small groups. Items that can help to stimulate memories are available from Age Concern and the Alzheimer's Society (contact details in Appendix 1).

People with dementia often appear to enjoy reminiscence therapy, although it probably does not prevent the memory from getting worse in the long run.

Can you explain what reality orientation is?

Reality orientation is a technique in which people caring for individuals with dementia take every opportunity to orientate them. For example, a member of staff in a hospital or nursing home may remind someone with dementia where they are and what time of day it is each time they meet. As part of this approach staff members would also correct someone with dementia when they make a mistake. Many people with dementia find this upsetting.

I am in charge of a nursing home and some of my residents disturb the others by shouting and screaming. I am aware of criticism of the over-use of drugs in nursing homes. Are there any other ways I can tackle this problem?

Sometimes people with dementia shout or scream because they are in pain or discomfort due to various causes (such as those given as causes of restlessness in the section 'Restlessness and agitation' in Chapter 7). When no cause can be identified, it may be possible to stop difficult behaviour without resort to drugs.

If the behaviour is precipitated by a particular event or situation, it may be possible to take action to avoid it. For example, if shouting occurs when someone is waiting for a meal, making sure that they are given their meal first may sometimes improve matters. If there is no obvious trigger, it may help to give the person with dementia more attention when they are not shouting or screaming rather than responding to them immediately they start to shout or scream. This has the effect of encouraging the more desirable behaviour rather than reinforcing the difficult behaviour. Your home's GP may be able to put you in touch with your local psychology service who could give advice about how to assess the problem and find solutions.

Our local hospital is raising money for a Snoezelen. What is this?

Snoezelens have now been installed in a number of hospitals, care homes and day centres. A Snoezelen is a special room designed to gently stimulate the senses while also helping agitated people to relax. There are comfortable places to sit, coloured moving lights and restful music. Some Snoezelens also have pleasant aromas. Snoezelens are thought to be a pleasant activity for some people with dementia.

COMPLEMENTARY MEDICINE

Might alternative or complementary therapies help someone with Alzheimer's disease?

There is no reason why a person with Alzheimer's disease should not try complementary therapies. There are many possible approaches, including homeopathy, osteopathy, acupuncture, massage, aromatherapy, Reiki and spiritual healing. Unfortunately, because of the nature of these treatments, they are often 'unproven' scientifically, but this should not stop you from seeking advice or trying them out.

One note of caution: if you do decide to try a form of complementary therapy, it is always wise to consult a practitioner who is accredited by a professional body. Further information is available from the Institute for Complementary Medicine (contact details in Appendix 1).

It is also important that you inform a patient's doctor what complementary medicines someone is taking, as there are instances where these can cause side effects or interact with other medicine.

What is Ginkgo biloba, *and is it true that it can help people with dementia?*

Ginkgo biloba is extracted from the gingko tree and has been used for centuries for treating various conditions. In some countries, such as Germany, it is widely used for many different conditions. It is not clear if it helps in dementia.

Ginkgo biloba does not need a prescription and is available over the counter from pharmacies and health food shops. It generally causes very few side effects but if you are taking any other medication, you should check with your doctor before taking ginkgo.

My wife has been diagnosed with Alzheimer's disease and I'd like her to see a spiritual healer. How do we go about this?

Spiritual healers, also known as contact healers or faith healers, see people with a wide variety of illnesses, including Alzheimer's disease. As with other complementary treatments, you would be wise to consult a practitioner who is bound by the professional code of conduct of a recognised organisation. There are several organisations of spiritual healers in the UK. Further information may be obtained from the Institute for Complementary Medicine or the National Federation of Spiritual Healers (contact details in Appendix 1).

13 | Research

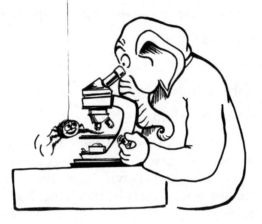

There is an enormous amount of research going on world wide into causes and cures of dementia. The need for research is urgent because people are living longer and the number of people with dementia is increasing. Dementia is a distressing illness and its effects are far-reaching. The need to care for people with dementia takes a toll both on individuals doing the caring and on governments providing the resources. This chapter does not include details of individual research projects as those that are successful will take many years to become widely available. It does, however, describe the main areas of research and how you can get involved.

RESEARCH OVERVIEW

What are the main areas of research into dementia at the present time?

The main areas of research at the moment include:

- trying to find the cause of different types of dementias;
- how Alzheimer's disease causes damage to the brain;
- trying to find simple tests;
- how the progression of dementia can be slowed down by drugs;
- how the behavioural changes can be treated;
- how carers can be helped.

Much has already been discovered about the changes that take place in the brains of people with various types of dementia. Much less is known about why these changes occur. Until researchers can find why these illnesses start, there is little hope of finding a cure.

Some of the most exciting discoveries in the last few years have been in drug treatments that may slow down the progression of the disease. A number of such drugs are now available (see the section 'Drug treatments' in Chapter 12) and much more research is being done to improve treatments for dementia.

Where can I get up-to-date, accurate information on research into Alzheimer's and other dementias?

Probably the best source of up-to-date information on dementia is the web (internet) if you have access to a computer with a modem.

Searching the internet using a phrase such as 'Alzheimer's disease' will identify thousands of websites, many of which contain inaccurate or misleading information. In order to ensure that the information you get from the internet is of high quality and accurate, try searching through the website 'www.intute.ac.uk'. Once there, go to the 'Health and Life Sciences' pages and then you can search for what you want. Intute filters out the poor quality information, but puts you in touch with good sites, such as those of the Department of Health and the Alzheimer's Society.

Alzheimer's societies in many countries provide regular newsletters that include articles on research topics written by researchers in the field. The Alzheimer's Society also produces easy-to-understand information sheets on new developments as they come through.

Newspapers, magazines, radio and television programmes quite often give coverage to research into Alzheimer's disease and other dementias. However, it is important to remember that not all the information they give is accurate, and there is a tendency for the popular press to make too much of apparently promising early research findings. All too often, the claims turn out to have been exaggerated or misplaced.

Where does the funding for medical research into diseases such as Alzheimer's disease come from?

There are three main sources of funding for medical research: the government (using revenue from taxation), pharmaceutical companies and charities.

In the UK, the government's contribution to medical research funding takes different forms. It includes money allocated to the National Health Service (NHS), the Medical Research Council (MRC), the Department of Health and also the universities (through the Department for Education and Skills). Government money finances most of the long-term infrastructure for medical research (including hospitals and university research departments), as well as providing money for specific medical research projects.

Pharmaceutical companies together contribute the largest share (in excess of 50%) of all medical research funding in the UK. Developing new drugs costs a great deal of money, but the profits from a successful drug for a common disease such as Alzheimer's disease are potentially enormous. Pharmaceutical companies fund research in their own laboratories and also often run drug trials (discussed later in this chapter) involving many researchers in centres around the country.

Charities, such as the Alzheimer's Society in England, also spend significant amounts of money on research each year. Charity money is generally spent on financing specific research projects, which are carefully selected for quality and effectiveness. In recent years, the Alzheimer's Society has funded research into improving the diagnosis, gene therapies and other treatment approaches in dementia.

Is there international collaboration of research into dementia as there is with AIDS?

Specific research projects into dementias tend to be locally or nationally based. However, the researchers involved in these projects belong to a wider scientific community. Scientists from many countries often come together at international conferences to share their ideas and present their research findings. Among the groups that organise such conferences are the International Psychogeriatric Association and Alzheimer's Disease International. Researchers also read medical journals published in other countries, and communicate with colleagues in other countries via the internet.

Despite a lot of media hype, it seems to me that not many new treatments for dementia ever see the light of day. Why is this?

Thousands of scientists around the world are working hard to find better treatments for dementia. When potentially good treatments are found, this is exciting news and they receive a lot of publicity in the media. However, many 'discoveries' are never heard of again, either because they don't work as well as was initially thought or because they are found to be unsafe. Even when a line of research does lead to a new treatment, such as the drug donepezil (Aricept) (see the section 'Drug treatments' in Chapter 12), there will always have been a research and trial period of several years between the initial research findings and the granting of a licence to make the drug available for use.

What processes must a drug go through before it becomes available for general use?

Before any drug can be made generally available, either on prescription or over the counter, it has to undergo numerous tests to make sure that it works and also that it is safe. Only a tiny proportion of the drugs that are under development ever become available for use by the general public.

If a drug is thought to be of potential use, it is first of all tested in the laboratory and then its safety is tested on healthy human volunteers. Following this, the drug may be given to selected patients taking part in carefully monitored drug trials. If extensive testing shows that a drug is both safe and useful, it will be approved by the European Medicines Agency and by the Medicines and Healthcare products Regulatory Agency (MHRA) in the UK. This may take many years from the first discovery of the drug.

Only after a drug has been approved for safety and effectiveness can a pharmaceutical company market it, or doctors prescribe it, to patients other than those in drug trials.

HELPING WITH RESEARCH

My husband has been told he's got dementia but that it is in an early stage. I have talked this through with him and we are keen to help research into a cure. What can be done?

To take part in a research study, your husband will need to meet various entry criteria. This usually means that:

- there must be no doubt about the diagnosis of dementia;

- the dementia is not at an advanced stage; and

- the person is otherwise medically quite fit.

It is probably worth talking first to your husband's GP. He or she may be able to put you in contact with a specialist at the local hospital, who may know about studies taking place in your area. Recently an organisation called the Dementia and Neurodegenerative Diseases Research Network was set up across the UK, intended to help scientists find people to take part in research. More information is available from the UK Clinical Research Network (website address in Appendix 1). Alternatively, the Alzheimer's Society or Alzheimer Scotland (contact details in Appendix 1) may have information about local trials.

Before helping out with any research, you and your husband should consider the following points:

- What is the research trying to find out?

- Can it help your husband directly, or just help others later?

- What time commitment is involved? (There are often very frequent visits to clinics, for example.)

- What tests will my husband (and I) have?

- Is there a chance that my husband will be given only a placebo (see the section 'Drug trials', next)?

- What happens when the trial ends? (For example, if the drug is benefiting your husband, can he continue with it?)

All medical research in the UK is very closely regulated and the people running the study should be happy to discuss these points with you and your husband. Even if you commit to a research study, you will be able to leave the trial at any time without having to give a reason.

My wife has been asked to take part in a study that involves having a brain scan. She is quite confused now and doesn't really understand what is being asked. I think the research is a good thing. Can I give consent for my wife?

It is possible to do research on people who are unable to give informed consent as long as certain safeguards are met. In Scotland the Adults with Mental Incapacity Act 2000 and in England and Wales the Mental Capacity Act 2005 have clarified what should be done. The researcher should inform you of the research project and ask you whether you think your wife should take part in the project and what her views would have been about the research when she was well. When speaking with the researcher, check that the study has been passed by an ethics committee.

DRUG TRIALS

What happens if we agree that my husband will help in a drug trial?

Drug trials are usually conducted at many sites throughout the country, so it should not be necessary to travel very far to take part. The usual procedure would be for you and your husband to go and see a doctor or other researcher involved with the trial. You will both probably be interviewed and asked to fill in a questionnaire. Your husband will then probably be given a thorough physical examination, a memory test, blood tests and perhaps a test of heart function.

If your husband is considered eligible for the trial, he will be given a supply of tablets. These may be either the new medication or a placebo (an inactive compound, usually a harmless sugar). Neither you nor your husband nor the researchers you see will know which tablets he receives. You will be given instructions about how many tablets your husband needs to take, and how often. It is important that you try to make sure that these instructions are followed.

You and your husband will then need to see the researcher regularly, usually for a period of at least 16 weeks, so that your husband's condition can be monitored. Your husband will probably need to have further blood tests and memory tests each time you see the researcher. You may be asked about how you think your husband is doing.

My husband is taking part in a study that is testing a new treatment for Alzheimer's disease. But I have not been told whether he is having the proper drug or the placebo. Why is this?

Your husband is in what is known as a placebo-controlled trial. In such trials, some of the participants are given the active drug, while others are given a placebo (an inactive compound, usually a harmless sugar) that looks exactly the same. Participants are not told whether they are being given the active drug or the placebo, because giving people this information can affect the results of the trial.

The trial will also be what is called a double-blind trial, meaning that the researchers you see will also not know which is which, because this knowledge might affect how they treat different participants and thus also affect the results of the trial.

The reason for giving some people a placebo when a new medication is under trial is that the actual participation in a trial can in itself lead to an improvement that may mistakenly be thought to be due to the drug.

My husband received a new drug while taking part in a clinical trial and seemed to be doing well. As the trial has now stopped, will it be possible for him to continue the drug?

To a great extent, the answer depends on the company that is conducting the trial. In some instances, patients who have done well with a particular drug will be able to continue taking it after the trial has finished. In other instances, this will not be possible, at least for the time being. If the trial in which your husband took part proves successful, your husband's doctor will, of course, be able to prescribe him the drug when it becomes generally available.

OTHER AREAS OF RESEARCH

What can genetic research tell us about the development of Alzheimer's disease, and how might this information be put to practical use?

Genetic research has already identified several genes that play a part in the development of Alzheimer's disease (discussed in the section 'Causes of Alzheimer's disease' in Chapter 2).

With the completion of the Human Genome Project, it is very likely that further genes which play a role will be identified in the future. It is also possible that further research will be able to discover how abnormal genes actually cause the disease or assist it to develop.

The first practical application of genetic research into the causes of Alzheimer's disease has been the development of a test (see the section 'Genetic tests' in Chapter 3) for the very rare forms of Alzheimer's disease that are passed on by a single gene. The potential usefulness of developing genetic tests for other forms of Alzheimer's disease seems less clear at present, especially in the absence of a cure for the disease.

Genetic testing may in the future decide who will get the most benefit from drugs designed to treat Alzheimer's disease or to identify types of Alzheimer's disease needing particular treatment.

In theory, it might be possible at some stage to replace or repair damaged genes, including those implicated in the development of Alzheimer's disease. However, research of this type is still very much in its infancy and practical results cannot be expected for many years yet.

Has any research been carried out into non-medical treatments for dementia?

There has been a certain amount of research into various non-medical treatments for dementia. For example, researchers have looked into the use of bright lights and music to calm people with agitated behaviour, the use of strong magnetic fields to try to improve memory, and the effects on the brain of physical and mental exercise. Some of the preliminary findings look promising, but more research is needed.

Is there any research into ways of helping carers to cope with looking after someone with dementia?

There has been a lot of research into how caring for someone with dementia affects the carer and how stress on the carer can be reduced. Research has found that, on the whole, carers do an excellent job despite having no formal training but that stress is often a major problem.

Caring for someone with dementia typically results in a major change in a carer's lifestyle. Despite this, many carers tend not to make full use of the practical and emotional support that is available to them from other family members, Social Services and carers' support groups. Researchers have found that practical assistance in the home, day care and respite care significantly reduce carer stress by allowing carers time for themselves. (See Chapter 9 for more information about getting help and support.)

The demands of caring for someone with dementia have been shown to result in an increased risk of physical problems and depression in some carers. To some extent, these problems can be reduced by having help from other members of the family, learning how to cope with problem behaviours, and receiving good support and helpful information from doctors, nurses and other professionals.

Glossary

Terms in *italics* in these definitions also appear as entries in the Glossary.

acetylcholine one of a group of chemicals known as *neurotransmitters*. Found throughout the brain, acetylcholine enables nerve cells to communicate with each other. In *Alzheimer's disease*, the levels of acetylcholine are lower than usual

AIDS abbreviation for Acquired Immune Deficiency Syndrome

Alzheimer's disease the most common type of *dementia*. It usually begins after the age of 65 and results in gradual, progressive loss of memory and other functions of the brain

amyloid a protein that is found in the brains of people with *Alzheimer's disease*. It is deposited throughout the brain in microscopic clumps called plaques. Its function is unknown and it may be the cause of the deterioration of brain function

anticholinergic drugs a term for drugs that reverse or inhibit the action of *acetylcholine* on nerve cells

anticholinesterase drugs also known as cholinesterase inhibitors, these *dementia drugs* stop the breakdown of *acetylcholine*. They may help to slow down the progression of *Alzheimer's disease* in some people. Examples include donepezil (Aricept) and galantamine (Reminyl)

antipsychotic drugs a range of *tranquillisers*, also known as neuroleptic drugs, that help to reduce symptoms of aggression. They may also be used for treating *hallucinations*. Examples include risperidone, olanzapine and quetiapine. These drugs have side effects and should be used with caution in people with *dementia*

Aricept the brand name for donepezil, a *dementia drug*

brain scan a general term to mean any investigation that produces pictures of the brain. A *CT scan* or *MRI scan* shows 'slices' through the brain. A *SPECT scan* shows the brain's blood supply

care home a name covering *nursing homes* (sometimes called 'care home (nursing)' and *residential homes* (sometimes called just 'care home'). Two-thirds of the people they currently look after have *dementia*

care manager a person from a *Social Services* department (or sometimes from *Community Health Services*) whose job it is to put together, monitor and review the care plan agreed after a *needs assessment* for *community care*

carer in the broadest sense, a carer is a person who provides help and support to another person, usually a relative or friend. More specifically, a carer is someone who looks after another person who needs help with daily living and who would not otherwise be able to live independently at home. The person who cares for a relative, friend or neighbour is often called a 'family carer'; a paid carer is usually called a 'care worker'

CAT scan abbreviation for Computed Axial Tomography scan. Another name for a *CT scan*

cerebral cortex the outer layers of the brain, involved in thinking, memory and the interpretation of perception or the senses

cerebrospinal fluid the fluid that surrounds the brain and spinal cord

cholinergic referring to *acetylcholine*. For example, a cholinergic *neurone* is a brain cell that contains the chemical acetylcholine

cholinesterase inhibitor an alternative name for an *anticholinesterase drug*

chromosomes microscopic thread-like structures that are present in all cells. They are collections of *genes*, which contain the genetic information that is transmitted from generation to generation

CJD (Creutzfeldt–Jakob disease) a very rare form of *dementia* caused by an infectious agent called a prion. As well as loss of memory, CJD commonly causes muscle jerking, blindness and problems with walking. Death occurs within a year or so

clinical trial an investigation, involving patients, that is designed to find out whether a new drug or other treatment is effective

cognitive tests tests that assess how well a person can think and how well his or her memory is working

cognitive therapy a treatment that involves getting a person to think differently about a problem or situation

Commission for Social Care Inspection the government body responsible for regulating and inspecting *care homes*

community care a term covering health and social care services delivered to people in the community, usually in their own home

Community Health Services or **Community Health Trusts** parts of the NHS, which provide health care in people's own homes or in local clinics and health centres

community mental health nurse a community-based nurse who is specially trained to look after the psychological needs of people living at home (formerly called community psychiatric nurse, or CPN)

complementary medicine an approach to health care that explores additions to conventional treatments. Acupuncture, *homeopathy*, aromatherapy and spiritual healing are examples of complementary therapies

confusion a state in which problems with memory and concentration impair the function of the mind

consultant a doctor who usually works from a hospital and who has specialist knowledge about a particular field of medicine. Consultants involved in the care of people with *dementia* include *geriatricians*, *neurologists* and *psychiatrists*

continuing care long-term care provided or paid for by the NHS. Continuing care of people with *dementia* has now been largely replaced by care in *care homes* paid for personally or by *Social Services*

CT scan a computed tomography scan. This is an X-ray scan that results in a series of pictures or 'slices' through the brain. Also known as a CAT (computed axial tomography) scan

day care the provision of day-time care in a *day centre*. Day care for people with *dementia* may involve practical help, such as with bathing, chiropody, etc., and also activities, such as *reminiscence therapy* and exercises

day centre a facility, run by a Health Authority, Social Services or a voluntary organisation, that provides *day care* for people who are unable to look after themselves. People attend the centre during the day and return home in the evenings

dehydration a state in which there is insufficient water in the body. It occurs when a person's fluid intake fails to balance fluid lost through sweating, vomiting or diarrhoea

dementia a term used to describe impairment of brain function, involving *memory*, thinking and concentration. Dementia usually becomes progressively worse, eventually making it impossible for someone to cope with living without help. There are many types of dementia, including *Alzheimer's disease, vascular dementia, Lewy body dementia* and *Pick's disease*

dementia drugs a term for drugs used to treat *dementia*. They include *anticholinesterase drugs*, and other drugs, such as *memantine* (Ebixa), which have a different mechanism of action. These drugs may slow down the progression of dementia in some people

depression an illness in which the main symptoms are feeling low, tearfulness and loss of enjoyment. Depression can affect sleep, appetite, motivation and concentration. It is treatable

diagnosis the process of identifying and naming a disease from a person's symptoms and signs. Getting a diagnosis may only involve talking with the doctor and having a physical examination. In other cases, special investigations may need to be done as well

disinhibition loss of the feelings of shame or embarrassment that normally help control a person's actions. Disinhibition results in inappropriate or improper behaviour

disorientation a state in which someone loses their awareness of time and place. For example, they may fail to recall the date or even the year, and may not be able to say where they are

donepezil the *generic* name of Aricept, a *dementia drug*

double-blind trial a type of *clinical trial* in which different groups of people are given a new treatment or a *placebo* or an established treatment. Neither the people in the trial nor those assessing the responses know which treatment any individual is given. This is to make sure that any improvement in a person's condition is not due simply to taking part in the trial

Enduring Power of Attorney (EPA) a legal document in which one person gave another the power to handle his or her financial affairs. Since October 2007, it is no longer possible to draw up an EPA as it has been replaced by a *Lasting Power of Attorney*. Existing EPAs are still valid, however

Exelon the brand name for rivastigmine, a *dementia drug*

frontal lobe dementia a *dementia* in which the disease process affects mainly the *frontal lobes* of the brain. Memory is affected less than in other dementias, but there may be major problems with loss of motivation and *disinhibition*

frontal lobes parts of the *cerebral cortex* situated at the front of the brain. This is the area of the brain that controls movement of the body. It is also involved in 'higher functions', such as planning, problem solving and initiative

galantamine the *generic* name of Reminyl, a type of *dementia drug*

generic a generic drug is a drug that is sold under its official medical name (its generic name, e.g. galantamine) rather than under a patented brand name (e.g. Reminyl)

genes material contained within the chromosomes. Genes carry the blueprint for the body: information that dictates how our bodies are built up, including the colour of our eyes and skin, how tall we are, our gender and many other details. Some genes have defects, or mutations, that cause disease

geriatrician a doctor who specialises in the treatment of physical illnesses in older people

hallucination a perception (hearing, seeing, smelling or feeling something) without an appropriate stimulus. For example, hearing voices when there is no one there. Hallucinations are quite common in people with *dementia*

HIV abbreviation for Human Immunodeficiency Virus

home care the provision of care workers to help look after people in their own homes, usually arranged by *Social Services*. These *home care assistants* generally provide personal care, such as help with washing and dressing, preparing meals and other activities of daily life

home care assistant a person who is paid to provide practical help, such as with shopping and cleaning and help getting up in the morning, to someone in their own home

home help a common name for *home care assistant*

homeopathy a branch of *complementary medicine* based on the principle that 'like cures like'. A homeopath will prescribe very dilute amounts of substances that, in larger quantities, would cause the same symptoms as the illness being treated

Huntington's disease also sometimes called Huntington's chorea, a disease in which mental deterioration is accompanied by involuntary twitching and muscle spasms

incontinence involuntary or inappropriate passing of urine or faeces. Help is available from continence advisers

Lasting Power of Attorney (LPA) a legal document in which one person gives another or others the power to handle his or her personal affairs. This can only be set up when the person giving it is mentally capable of understanding what he or she is doing. See also *Enduring Power of Attorney*

laxative a medicine that treats constipation either by providing more fibre or by stimulating the bowel

Lewy body dementia a type of *dementia* in which abnormal collections of protein, called Lewy bodies, occur in the brain. People with Lewy body dementia typically show more variation in their mental abilities from day to day than is usual with other dementias

memantine a *dementia drug* (brand name Ebixa) that works by altering chemicals, called NMDA receptors, in the brain. It may slow down the progression of *dementia* in some people with moderate to severe *Alzheimer's disease*

memory the retention in the mind of information that may be recalled later

Mental Capacity Act 2005 an Act of Parliament that provides safeguards for people who lack 'mental capacity' (i.e. are not able to decide things for themselves)

Mental Health Act 1983 an Act of Parliament that governs the treatment and care of individuals incapacitated by mental illness. A section of the Act allows a person to be compulsorily detained and treated in hospital. Different Acts apply in Scotland and Northern Ireland

mentally incapacitated being unable, through mental disorder, to take charge of financial and other affairs

MRI scan abbreviation for Magnetic Resonance Imaging scan. A type of *brain scan* that creates pictures using a powerful magnetic field instead of X-rays

multi-disciplinary referring to a team made up of professionals from different specialities, typically including doctors, nurses, *psychologists, social workers* and *occupational therapists*

multi-infarct dementia another name for *vascular dementia*

needs assessment the process by which *Social Services* and health professionals assess the services that a person should be provided with under local *community care* provisions

neuroleptic drugs another name for *antipsychotic drugs*

neurologist a doctor who specialises in the diagnosis, treatment and management of diseases of the nervous system

neurone a nerve cell

neurotransmitters a group of chemicals in the brain that enable nerve cells to communicate with each other. Groups of adjacent nerve cells tend to use the same neurotransmitter. Examples include *acetylcholine*, serotonin and dopamine

nursing home a *care home* that is required by law to employ qualified nurses and to provide 24-hour nursing care. (Also called 'care home (nursing)'.)

occupational therapist a person who can advise on ways of helping someone to maintain their skills and independence for as long as possible. They can also advise on aids in the person's home

Parkinson's disease a chronic (long-term) disease of the nervous system that is characterised by slowness of movements, a tremor and an expressionless face. Some people with Parkinson's disease also develop *dementia*

Patient Advice and Liaison Service (PALS) a service that takes up complaints with the local hospital or GP on behalf of patients. PALS also acts as a link between patients and the providers of health care

PET scan abbreviation for Positron Emission Tomography scan. A sophisticated brain scan that is able to look at the brain in great detail

physiotherapist a person trained to perform and advise on physical treatments for joint and muscle problems

Pick's disease a rare *dementia* that commonly affects younger people than people with *Alzheimer's disease*. It affects language and personality before there is any significant change in *memory*

placebo the name given in *double-blind trials* to the non-active substance with which an active drug is being compared. It is a 'dummy' version of the drug, identical in appearance to the drug being tested

primary progressive aphasia a condition in which people may progressively lose their speech altogether

psychiatrist a doctor who specialises in the diagnosis and treatment of mental illness

psychogeriatrician a doctor who specialises in the diagnosis and treatment of mental illness in older people

psychologist someone with training in psychology, the study of behaviour. Clinical psychologists assess and treat people who have mental disorders

psychotherapy a 'talking therapy' that can help people to understand their own feelings and therefore feel more confident to deal with them

reality orientation a psychological treatment in which every opportunity is taken to make people with *dementia* aware of the time, where they are and the world around them

receiver someone appointed to take responsibility for handling the financial affairs of a person with *dementia* when that person is no longer able to do this for him- or herself. The receiver may be a close relative, a friend, the local authority or a solicitor

reminiscence therapy a therapy that aims to stimulate people's memories by means of films, pictures, music, etc., from their past

Reminyl the brand name for galantamine, a *dementia drug*

residential home the common name for a *care home*, which supplies accommodation for people who are no longer able to manage everyday tasks or to maintain an independent home of their own. In general, residential homes take people who need less care than is provided in a *nursing home*

respite care a facility or resource that allows *carers* to have a break. Respite care may be provided in a *residential home* or *nursing home*, in a person's own home or with another family

rivastigmine the *generic* name for Exelon, a *dementia drug*

sedative drugs drugs used to reduce symptoms of anxiety and agitation and to help people sleep. Sedative drugs can increase confusion in people with *dementia*

semantic dementia the person can't find the right words, or loses all the meaning for words that were previously familiar to them

sheltered housing units where people can live independently but where there is a warden on call who can offer a certain amount of supervision. Some support services may also be available

side effects the unwanted effects that occur in addition to the desired therapeutic effects of a drug. Most drugs have some side effects. These will vary from person to person and commonly disappear when the body becomes used to a particular drug

Snoezelen a special room designed to gently stimulate the senses and to calm people who are agitated

Social Services a local government (local authority) department responsible for the non-medical welfare and care of people in need. Social Services departments organise *needs assessments* for people with *dementia* and provide services under *community care* provisions

social worker a professional who can offer advice on practical matters in connection with finances, *day care* and accommodation. A social worker will look at problems in the context of the family and the community. Some specialise in mental illness

SPECT scan a Single Photon Emission Computed Tomography scan. A highly technical investigation similar to a *PET scan*

stroke a result of a haemorrhage in the brain or of a blood clot in an artery of the brain, leading to paralysis of part or all of one side of the body, or loss of speech, or loss of consciousness or death. The paralysis may be sudden or gradual in onset

support group a group, also known as a self-help group, that aims to provide mutual support for its members. A support group gives *carers* an opportunity to share their feelings, problems and information with other people undergoing similar experiences

thyroid a gland in the neck that produces a chemical known as thyroid hormone. This hormone is essential to the workings of the body. Thyroid hormone deficiency is a rare cause of *dementia*

tranquillisers drugs used to help people who are very anxious. These drugs can cause increased confusion in people with *dementia*

vascular dementia a type of *dementia* associated with problems affecting the circulation of blood to the brain, such as may result from a series of small *strokes*

vitamins chemical compounds essential to health that are found in many foods. Vitamin deficiency is a rare cause of *dementia*

voluntary organisation any organisation run on a not-for-profit basis. Many of the people who work for voluntary organisations do so without payment

Appendix 1: Useful addresses

Age Concern England
Astral House
1268 London Road
London SW16 4ER
Helpline: 0800 00 99 66
Tel: 020 8765 7200
Website: www.ageconcern.org.uk
*Researches into the needs of older
people and is involved in policy
making. Provides advice on a range of
subjects for people over 50. Publishes
books and offers services via local
branches.*

Age Concern Scotland
Causewayside House
160 Causewayside
Edinburgh EH9 1PP
Helpline: 0845 125 9732
Tel: 0845 833 0200
Website: www.ageconcernscotland.org.uk
As Age Concern England.

Age Concern Cymru
Units 13 & 14 Neptune Court
Vanguard Way
Cardiff CF24 5PJ
Tel: 029 2043 1555
Website: www.accymru.org.uk
As Age Concern England.

Age Concern Northern Ireland
3 Lower Crescent
Belfast BT7 1NR
Tel: 028 9024 5729
Website: www.ageconcernni.org
As Age Concern England.

Alzheimer's Disease International
64 Great Suffolk Street
London SE1 0BL
Tel: 020 7981 0880
Website: www.adi.alz.co.uk
*Umbrella organisation for Alzheimer's
associations around the world.*

**Alzheimer Scotland – Action
on Dementia**
22 Drumsheugh Gardens
Edinburgh EH3 7RN
Helpline: 0808 808 3000
Tel: 0131 243 1453
Website: www.alzscot.org.uk
*Provides advice, support and local
services in Scotland for people with
dementia and their carers.*

Alzheimer Society of Ireland
43 Northumberland Avenue
Dun Laoghaire
Co Dublin, Ireland
Helpline: 1800 341 341
Tel: 00 353 1 2846616
Website: www.alzheimer.ie
Aims to maximise quality of life by
providing services and information for
people affected by Alzheimer's disease
and other dementias.

Alzheimer's Society
Devon House
St Katharine's Way
London E1W 1JK
Helpline: 0845 300 0336
Tel: 020 7423 3500
Website: www.alzheimers.org.uk
Care and research charity supplying
information and support for people
with dementia and their carers.

Quality and Information Team
Alzheimer's Society
Email:
to order publications:
pubsorders@alzheimers.org.uk
Dementia Knowledge Centre:
knowledgecentre@alzheimers.org.uk

Alzheimer's Society,
Northern Ireland
86 Eglantine Avenue
Belfast BT9 6EU
Tel: 028 9066 4100
Website:
www.alzheimers.org.uk/NIreland/Belfast
As for Alzheimer's Society.

Alzheimer's Society,
Wales
3rd Floor
Baltic House
Mount Stuart Square
Cardiff CF10 5FH
Tel: 029 2048 0953
Website: www.alzheimers.org.uk
As for Alzheimer's Society.

Benefits Agency
see Department for Work
and Pensions

Benefits Enquiry Line (BEL)
Freephone for England, Scotland
and Wales: 0800 882 200
Freephone for Northern Ireland:
0800 220 674
Website: www.dss.gov.uk
For information on state benefits for
people with disabilities and their
carers.

Carers Association Ireland
Prior's Orchard
John's Quay
Kilkenny, Ireland
Helpline: 1800 240 724
Tel: 00 353 056 772 1424/
    056 773 532
Website: www.carersireland.com
*Lobbies and advocates on behalf of
carers in Ireland. Offers home respite
service, information, training unit and
careline.*

Carers UK
20–25 Glasshouse Yard
London EC1A 4JT
Helpline: 0808 808 7777
Tel: 020 7490 8818
Website: www.carersuk.org
*Offers information and support to all
people who care for others with
medical or other problems.*

Christian Council on Ageing
(for enquiries/correspondence)
Dr Mike Lewis
47 Alard Close
Northampton
Northants NN3 5LZ
Tel: 01604 403578
Email: enquiries@ccoa.org.uk
Website: www.ccoa.org.uk
*Campaigns on behalf of older
Christians. Publishes books and
provides pastoral care within the
church and wider community.*

Citizens Advice Bureaux
Addresses and telephone numbers
of local offices are listed in the *Phone
Book*, and in *Yellow Pages* under
'Counselling and Advice'.

CJD Support Network
PO Box 346
Market Drayton
Shropshire TF9 4WN
Helpline: 01630 673 973
Website: www.cjdsupport.net
*Provides help and support for people
with all strains of CJD, their carers
and concerned professionals. Runs a
national helpline and can help families
in financial need.*

**Commission for
Social Care Inspection**
33 Greycoat Street
London SW1 2QF
Customer Services Helpline:
0845 015 0120
Website: www.csci.org.uk
*The official body regulating care homes
and agencies that provide nurses or
care workers who carry out personal
tasks.*

Counsel and Care
Twyman House
16 Bonny Street
London NW1 9PG
Helpline: 0845 300 7585
Tel: 020 7241 8555
Website: www.counselandcare.org.uk
Voice for all older people and their families. Advises on a number of issues, including community care, welfare benefits and hospital discharge.

Court of Protection
see Public Guardianship Office

Crossroads Care
Attendants Schemes
10 Regent Place
Rugby
Warwickshire CV21 2PN
Tel: 0845 450 0350
Website: www.crossroads.org.uk
Aims to improve the lives of carers by giving practical support and providing a paid, trained person to offer respite care in the home.

Cruse Bereavement Care
PO Box 800
Richmond
Surrey TW9 1RG
Helpline: 0844 477 9400
Tel: 020 8939 9530
Website: www.crusebereavementcare.org.uk
Aims to promote the well-being of bereaved people by providing one-to-one counselling and support.

Offers literature and practical advice and runs training in bereavement counselling for professionals.

Dementia Relief Trust
see For Dementia

Department for Work and Pensions
The address and telephone number of your local office will be in the *Phone Book* and in *Yellow Pages* under 'Social Services'.

Dignity in Dying
13 Prince of Wales Terrace
London W8 5PG
Tel: 0870 777 7868
Website: www.dignityindying.org.uk
Promotes patient choice at end of life and is campaigning for a change in the law to protect patients' rights. Leading supplier of 'living wills' in the UK.

Disability Alliance
Universal House
88–94 Wentworth Street
London E1 7SA
Tel: 020 7247 8776
Website: www.disabilityalliance.org
Information and support for people with disabilities and their carers.

DVLA (Driver and Vehicle Licensing Authority)
Medical Branch
Longview Road
Morriston
Swansea SA99 1TU
Helpline: 0870 600 0301
Website: www.dvla.gov.uk
Government office providing advice for drivers with special needs.

Elderly Accommodation Council
3rd Floor, 89 Albert Embankment
London SE1 7TP
Tel: 020 7820 1343
Website: www.housingcare.org
A source of information on all forms of accommodation for older people.

For Dementia
(formerly **Dementia Relief Trust**)
6 Camden High Street
London NW1 0JH
Helpline: 0845 257 9406
Tel: 020 7874 7210
Website: www.fordementia.org.uk
Focuses on providing specialist dementia nurses who can offer practical advice, emotional support and skills to families and carers of people with dementia.

Health Authority
The address and telephone number of your local Health Authority will be in the *Phone Book* and in *Yellow Pages* under 'Health Authority and Services'.

Human BSE Foundation
Matfen Court
Chester Le Street
County Durham DH2 2TX
Tel: 0191 389 4157
Website: www.hbsef.org
Offers support and up-to-date information to people with human BSE and their relatives, friends and care providers.

Huntington's Disease Association
1 London Bridge
London SE1 9BG
Tel: 020 7022 1950
Website: www.hda.org.uk
Offers support and understanding to anyone affected by Huntington's disease. Has a network of regional care advisers who provide information, workshops and educational services.

Incontact: Action on Incontinence
SATRA Innovation Park
Rockingham Road
Kettering
Northants NN16 9JH
Tel: 0870 770 3246
Website: www.incontact.org
Provides useful information and support for adults affected by bladder and bowel problems.

Institute for Complementary Medicine
PO Box 194
London SE16 7QZ
Tel: 020 7237 5165
Website: www.i-c-m.org.uk
Source of information on the safe practice of complementary medicine and a register of accredited practitioners and therapists near you.

Intute
www.intute.ac.uk
A free online service provided by a network of UK universities and partners. Once there, go to 'Health and Life Sciences' for reliable information.

Jewish Care
221 Golders Green Road
London NW11 9DQ
Helpline: 020 8922 2222
Website: www.jewishcare.org
Social care, personal support and residential homes for Jewish people.

Law Centre
The address and telephone number of your local Law Centre will be in the *Phone Book* and in *Yellow Pages* under 'Legal Services'.
Website: www.lawcentres.org.uk

MIND (National Association for Mental Health)
Granta House
15–19 Broadway, Stratford
London E15 4BQ
Helpline: 0845 766 0163
Tel: 020 8519 2122
Website: www.mind.org.uk
Mental health organisation working for a better life for anyone experiencing mental distress. Offers information and support via local branches.

National Council for Palliative Care
The Fitzpatrick Building
188–194 York Way
London N7 9AS
Tel: 020 7697 1520
Website: www.ncpc.org.uk
Promotes the extension and improvement of palliative care services for all people with life-threatening and life-limiting conditions.

National Federation of Spiritual Healers
Old Manor Farm Studio
Church Street
Sunbury-on-Thames
Middlesex TW16 6RG
Tel: 01932 783164
Website: www.nfsh.org.uk
Provides training for those who wish to become spiritual healers.

NHS Choices
www.nhs.uk
NHS website giving a range of information. Among other things, you can use it to find GP practices in your area.

Parkinson's Disease Society (PDS)

National Office
215 Vauxhall Bridge Road
London SW1V 1EJ
Helpline: 0808 800 0303
Tel: 020 7931 8080
Website: www.parkinsons.org.uk
Provides information and support for people with Parkinson's disease and their carers. Offers advice on living with Parkinson's and the drug, surgery and therapy options available.

Pick's Disease Support Group

www.pdsg.org.uk
Information and support for carers of people with Pick's disease. The website doesn't give a contact address but does give contact details for committee members in different areas of the UK.

Public Guardianship Office

Archway Tower
2 Junction Road
London N19 5SZ
Tel: 0845 330 2900
Website: www.guardianship.gov.uk
Responsible for providing services that promote the financial and social well-being of people with mental incapacity.

Quit

Tel: 0800 00 22 00
To get help with stopping smoking.

RADAR (Royal Association for Disability and Rehabilitation)

12 City Forum
125 City Road
London EC1V 8AF
Tel: 020 7250 3222
Textphone: 020 7250 4119
Website: www.radar.org.uk
Sells special key to access locked public toilets for the disabled.

Relate

Herbert Gray College
Little Church Street
Rugby
Warwickshire CV21 3AP
Helpline: 0845 456 1310
Tel: 01788 573241
Website: www.relate.org.uk
Offers relationship counselling via local branches, and publishes information on health, sexual, self-esteem, depression, bereavement and marriage issues.

Relatives and Residents Association

24 The Ivories
6–18 Northampton Street
London N1 2HY
Helpline: 020 7359 8136
Tel: 020 7359 8148
Website: www.relres.org
Offers support and advice for older relatives and friends of people in care homes or hospital long-term.

Samaritans

Tel: 08457 90 90 90

Website: www.samaritans.org.uk

Offers 24-hour helpline for people needing to talk. Also available by personal visit, by letter or by email.
By personal visit: see the Phone Book *for your local branch*
By letter: Chris, PO Box 9090, Stirling FK8 2SA (remember to give your address if you want a reply)
By email: jo@samaritans.org.uk

Social security

The address and telephone number of your local office will be in the *Phone Book* (probably under 'Jobcentre Plus').

Stroke Association

Stroke House

240 City Road

London EC1V 2PR

Helpline: 0845 303 3100

Website: www.stroke.org.uk

Offers comprehensive information and advice about stroke, with community services around the country. A major funder of stroke research.

Terrence Higgins Trust

314–320 Grays Inn Road

London WC1X 8DP

Helpline: 0845 1221 200

Tel: 020 7812 1600

Website: www.tht.org.uk

Provides information and advice on AIDS, HIV and sexual health. Can assist with housing, treatment, welfare, employment and legal matters.

UK Clinical Research Network

www.ukcrn.org.uk

Website giving information about research projects.

United Kingdom Home Care Association

Group House, 2nd Floor

52 Sutton Court Road

Sutton

Surrey SM1 4SL

Helpline: 020 8288 5291

Tel: 020 8288 5291

Website: www.ukhca.co.uk

Association of independent sector providers of private nursing care to people in their own homes. Can supply information and lists of organisations adhering to an approved code of practice.

Vitalise (formerly Winged Fellowship Trust)

12 City Forum

250 City Road

London EC1V 8AF

Tel: 0845 345 1972

Website: www.vitalise.org.uk

Provides holidays and respite care for disabled people and their carers.

Appendix 2: Some other reading
including CDs, DVDs and videos

The Alzheimer's Society produces a monthly newsletter and a wide range of practical information and advice sheets about all aspects of dementia and living with dementia. See Appendix 1 for contact details.
See also the websites listed at the end of Appendix 1.

ALZHEIMER'S DISEASE AND DEMENTIA

Dementia: diagnosis and management in primary care, Tools for Diagnosis, published by the Alzheimer's Society, London, 2007 [CD-ROM]
Understanding Vascular Dementia, published by the Alzheimer's Society, London, 2005
Your Guide to Alzheimer's Disease, by Alistair Burns, published by Hodder Arnold, London, 2005

LIVING WITH DEMENTIA

I'm Told I have Dementia: what you can do ... who you can turn to, published by the Alzheimer's Society, London, 2000
Listening to the Experts, published by Alzheimer Scotland – Action on Dementia, Edinburgh, 2005 [VHS video and DVD]
Memory Handbook: a practical guide to living with memory problems, published by the Alzheimer's Society, London, 2006

CARING

Caring for the Person with Dementia: a handbook for families and other carers, published by the Alzheimer's Society, London, 2002
Disability Rights Handbook, published by the Disability Alliance, London, annually
Help for Caregivers: practical tips on how to care for a person with dementia, published by Alzheimer's Disease International with the World Health

Organization, London, 2000 [available online (www.adi.alz.co.uk) in
English and Spanish and in print in Arabic, Chinese, Danish, Hebrew,
Hindi, Japanese, Russian and Serbian]

Making Difficult Decisions: the experience of caring for someone with dementia,
published by the Alzheimer's Society, London, 2005

*The 36-hour Day: a family guide to caring for people with Alzheimer's disease,
other dementias, and memory loss in later life*, 4th edition, by Nancy L
Mace, published by Johns Hopkins University Press, Baltimore MD,
2006

Your Rights to Money Benefits, by Sally West, published by Age Concern
Books, London, annually

Your Rights to Healthcare, 2nd edition, by Lorna Easterbrook, published by
Age Concern Books, London, 2007

RESEARCH

Alzheimer's Disease, by Paul Dash and Nicole Villemarette-Pittman,
published by Demos Medical Publishing, New York NY, 2005

British Medical Journal. For articles about up-to-date information on
dementia treatment, see the website www.besttreatments.com

Dementia: your questions answered, by Jeremy Brown and Jonathan Hillam,
published by Churchill Livingstone, Oxford, 2004

*Dementia UK: a report into the prevalence and cost of dementia, prepared by the
Personal Social Services Research Unit (PSSRU) at the London School of
Economics and the Institute of Psychiatry at King's College London, for the
Alzheimer's Society*, published by the Alzheimer's Society, London, 2007

BIOGRAPHY, AUTOBIOGRAPHY AND NOVELS

Alzheimer's from the Inside Out, by Richard Taylor, published by Health
Professions Press, Baltimore MD, 2007

Dancing with Dementia: my story of living positively with dementia, by
Christine Bryden, published by Jessica Kingsley Publishers, London,
2005

In Memory of Memories: experience of living with dementia, published by the
Alzheimer's Society, London, 2003

Rough Music, by Patrick Gale, published by Flamingo, London, 2001

Scar Tissue, by Michael Ignatieff, published by Chatto & Windus, London,
1993

Tangles and Starbursts: living with dementia, by Julia Darling and Sharon
   Bailey, published by the Alzheimer's Society, North Tyneside Branch,
   2001

YOUNGER PEOPLE WITH DEMENTIA

*The Alzheimer's Society Guide to Improving Services for Younger People with
   Dementia: planning and delivery guidelines for health professionals*,
   published by the Alzheimer's Society, London, 2007
*Ready or Not: a survey of services available in the UK for younger people with
   dementia 2005–2006*, published by the Alzheimer's Society, London,
   2006

FOR CHILDREN

About my Grandfather . . . About my Grandmother, published by the
   Alzheimer's Society, London, 2004 [VHS video and DVD]
Mile-high Apple Pie, by Laura Langston and Lindsey Gardiner, published
   by the Bodley Head, London, 2004
The Milk's in the Oven, by Lizi Hann, published by the Mental Health
   Foundation/Alzheimer Scotland – Action on Dementia, Edinburgh,
   2005
Need to Know about Alzheimer's Disease, by Jim McGuigan, published by
   Heinemann, Oxford, 2004

Index

Have you found *Alzheimer's and other Dementias: Answers at your fingertips* useful and practical? If so, you may be interested in other books from Class Publishing.

Type 2 Diabetes:
Answers at your fingertips £14.99
Dr Charles Fox and Dr Anne Kilvert

The latest edition of our bestselling reference guide on diabetes has now been split into two books covering the two distinct forms of the disease. These books maintain the popular question-and-answer format to provide practical advice for patients on every aspect of living with the condition.

> *'I have no hesitation in commending this book.'* – Sir Steve Redgrave, Vice President, Diabetes UK

Stroke:
Answers at your fingertips £17.99
Dr Anthony Rudd, Penny Irwin and Bridget Penhale

This essential guidebook tells you all about strokes – and, most importantly, how to recover from them.

As well as providing clear explanations of the medical processes, tests and treatments, the book is full of practical advice, including recuperation plans. You will find it inspiring.

Dump Your Toxic Waist!
Lose inches, beat diabetes
and stop that heart attack £14.99
Dr Derek Cutting

The easy, drug-free and medically accurate way to cut dramatically your risk of having a heart attack. Even if you already have heart disease, you can halt or even reverse its progress by following Dr Cutting's simple steps. Don't be a victim – take action now!

> *'Highly recommended.'*
> Michael Livingston, Director, HEART UK

Heart Health:
Answers at your fingertips £14.99
Dr Graham Jackson

This practical handbook, written by a leading cardiologist, answers all your questions about heart conditions. It tells you all about you and your heart and how to keep your heart healthy – or, if it has already been affected by heart disease, how to make it as strong as possible.

> *'Those readers who want to know more about the various treatments for heart disease will be much enlightened.'* – Dr James Le Fanu, *The Daily Telegraph*

High Blood Pressure:
Answers at your fingertips £14.99
Dr Tom Fahey, Professor Deirdre Murphy with Dr Julian Tudor Hart

The authors use all their years of experience as blood pressure experts to answer your questions on high blood pressure, in order to give you the information you need to bring your blood pressure down – and keep it down.

> *'Readable and comprehensive information'* – Dr Sylvia McLaughlan, Director General, The Stroke Association

Beating Depression £17.99
Dr Stefan Cembrowicz and Dr Dorcas Kingham

Depression is one of most common illnesses in the world – affecting up to one in four people at some time in their lives. This book shows sufferers and their families that they are not alone, and offers tried-and-tested techniques for overcoming depression.

> *'All you need to know about depression, presented in a clear, concise and readable way.'* – Ann Dawson, World Health Organization

PRIORITY ORDER FORM

Cut out or photocopy this form and send it (post free in the UK) to:

Class Publishing   **Tel: 01256 302 699**
FREEPOST 16705   **Fax: 01256 812 558**
Macmillan Distribution
Basingstoke RG21 6ZZ

Please send me urgently   *Post included*
(tick below)   *price per copy (UK only)*

☐ **Alzheimer's and other Dementias: Answers at your fingertips**
(ISBN 978 1 85959 148 2)   £17.99

☐ **Type 2 Diabetes: Answers at your fingertips** (ISBN 978 1 85959 176 5)   £17.99

☐ **Stroke: Answers at your fingertips** (ISBN 978 1 85959 113 0)   £20.99

☐ **Dump Your Toxic Waist!** (ISBN 978 1 85959 191 8)   £17.99

☐ **Heart Health: Answers at your fingertips** (ISBN 978 1 85959 157 4)   £20.99

☐ **High Blood Pressure: Answers at your fingertips** (ISBN 978 1 85959 090 4)   £17.99

☐ **Beating Depression** (ISBN 978 1 85959 150 5)   £20.99

TOTAL _____

Easy ways to pay

Cheque: I enclose a cheque payable to Class Publishing for £ _____

Credit card: Please debit my   ☐ Mastercard   ☐ Visa   ☐ Amex

Number _____ Expiry date _____

Name _____

My address for delivery is _____

_____

Town _____ County _____ Postcode _____

Telephone number (*in case of query*) _____

Credit card billing address if different from above _____

_____

Town _____ County _____ Postcode _____

Class Publishing's guarantee: remember that if, for any reason, you are not satisfied with these books, we will refund all your money, without any questions asked. Prices and VAT rates may be altered for reasons beyond our control.